The Blood Thinner Cure

The Blood Thinner Cure

A Revolutionary Seven-Step Lifestyle Plan for Stopping Heart Disease and Stroke

Kenneth R. Kensey, M.D., with Carol A. Turkington

CB
CONTEMPORARY BOOKS

Library of Congress Cataloging-in-Publication Data

Kensey, Kenneth R.
   The blood thinner cure: a revolutionary seven-step lifestyle plan for stopping heart disease and stroke / Kenneth R. Kensey, Carol A. Turkington.
      p.   cm.
   Includes index.
   ISBN 0-8092-9841-4
      1. Arteriosclerosis—Prevention.   2. Coronary heart disease—Etiology.
   3. Cerebrovascular disease—Etiology.   I. Turkington, Carol.   II. Title.
   RC692.K46   2001
   616.1'3605—dc21   00-64481

This publication is intended to provide accurate and authoritative information on the subject matter covered. It is sold with the understanding that the publisher is not engaged in providing professional medical services. Any use of the information in this book is at the reader's discretion. The author and publisher specifically disclaim any and all liability arising directly or indirectly from the use or application of any information contained in this book. If professional medical advice or other expert assistance is required, the services of a competent professional should be sought.

Cover design by Jeanette Wojtyla
Author photograph by Pam Helser & Associates Photography
Interior design by Precision Graphics

Published by Contemporary Books
A division of NTC/Contemporary Publishing Group, Inc.
4255 West Touhy Avenue, Lincolnwood (Chicago), Illinois 60712-1975 U.S.A.
Printed in the United States of America
International Standard Book Number: 0-8092-9841-4
01   02   03   04   05   06   LB   14   13   12   11   10   9   8   7   6   5   4   3   2   1

Contents

Part 3.   Special Populations

Acknowledgments

I want to thank the thousands of scientists and physicians who have dedicated so much time and effort to identifying all the risk factors for atherosclerosis. Without these pieces of the puzzle, the understanding of this disease from a mechanical perspective would never have been possible.

Introduction

When I met Harry in 1987, he had already had a balloon angioplasty on his leg in addition to an earlier triple bypass. I knew that his prognosis wasn't good: he was overweight, he had diabetes, and he'd been a smoker most of his life. I felt for this man, especially since he tried to be so stoic and upbeat in the face of his problems. When he came to me for checkups, my questions were always answered with: "Fine, Doc, doin' just fine." I prayed for the best and hoped Harry was right, but I suspected he was wrong. Over the next five years, he endured more balloon angioplasties, bypasses in both legs, amputation, strokes, heart attack, and another heart bypass—and a final heart attack that ended his life.

Stories like this are all too common in the life of a cardiologist. In fact, it was patients like Harry that helped fuel my desire to become a cardiologist, as well as my obsession with finding the true cause of vascular disease.

My passionate interest in understanding the true cause of atherosclerosis (blocked or clogged arteries) stems from a profound sense of frustration. In the twenty years since I was a resident practicing internal medicine in Kalamazoo, Michigan, I have watched the disease claim far too many lives. I've watched far too many brilliant doctors spending their time and money trying to battle the end stages of the disease—and having their own hearts broken in the process. Bypasses, balloon angioplasty, and stents represent a Band-Aid approach to atherosclerosis.

To most people, the word *bypass* may suggest a just-in-time solution to a life-threatening problem that will save them from future heart attacks. Unfortunately, nothing could be further from the truth.

The fact is that of the 350,000 heart bypass procedures performed in the United States each year, 70,000 of them are being done for the second time because the arteries have become blocked again. Eight percent of patients having their second bypass surgery will die from the surgery itself. Among those who don't die, about a third find that their arteries clog up again within six months; in almost all patients, the arteries will completely close off again within ten years, even with modifications in diet and lifestyle.

Stopping bypass surgery has been my primary concern for the last several decades, along with getting to the root of what really causes atherosclerosis in the first place. I always knew that if I could find the cause, doctors could treat the disease before it began instead of having to deal with its devastating end stages.

Back in the 1970s, as a resident I was especially fond of the elderly folks who make up the main population of heart attack and stroke victims. Their stories reminded me of my folks and family friends and neighbors back home in the farm belt of Ohio. Sometimes I sat by their bedsides for just a few extra minutes, knowing that my presence and caring gave as much comfort as my medical knowledge.

And there was the rub: I didn't have the medical knowledge to save people from the devastation of cardiovascular disease—no one did. Yet, so often, families seemed to accept the onset of atherosclerosis as a sad but natural and unchangeable end-of-life sequence of events. Why did they accept cardiovascular disease as inevitable? They didn't think of cancer that way.

I hated seeing patients going to bypass surgery. This painful and dangerous process involves cutting open a patient's chest, stopping the heart, and taking a vein from the leg to create a detour around the blocked artery. It wasn't uncommon for a patient to have four or five arteries treated at the same time in this way. Worst of all, this procedure didn't cure the problem; it just bought the patient some time. *It did not stop the disease.*

I was not so gracious in the face of defeat. In fact, I couldn't accept the idea that there was no better way to treat this disease or that its origins must always remain elusive. I was determined, somehow, to find a better way.

Long before my fellowship in cardiology, I'd been obsessed with trying to find a device that would remove the debris that accumulated in the arteries—some type of rotary catheter that would actually go in and unplug the blockage, much the way a plumber opens a blocked pipe in your bathroom. At the time, this idea conflicted with the established viewpoint that if you could break up the artery blockage, the debris would simply cause blocks further down the arteries. My idea was considered crazy, but I was a man with a dream and a profound sense of mission. I went to Saint Luke's Hospital at Iowa University and took a job in an emergency room; the predictable schedule gave me time to do research. During these hours, I toiled in the maintenance department at the university, trying to create a spinning device that would do the job I envisioned.

When I realized I needed help, I gathered engineers and consultants and built some prototypes. Shortly thereafter, I left Saint Luke's to accept a cardiology fellowship at Michael Reese Hospital in Chicago, where I was given the lab space to work on my artery catheter. I spent hours in the morgue, studying the ravages of atherosclerosis at close range.

The thing that struck me most forcefully was the rocklike solidity of what had once been pliable, living arterial tissue. Strong enough to deflect a surgical instrument, the arteries were so stiff that they reminded me of radiator pipes. I knew that this unnatural hardness had been there while the body had been alive and that in this hardness lay the cause of death.

What did it mean, that it was only the arteries, never any nearby veins, that showed this hardening—and always the same ones: the aorta and the coronary and carotid arteries, as well as the large femoral artery running down the leg. What was the possible connection? Why was I seeing bodies that had lost legs, but never hands, to atherosclerosis? Why was the disease so common in only certain specific sites?

The sound and the feel of those hardened arteries never left me. In the shadowed landscapes of my dreams, they would surface, apparently with some message, if only I could decipher it. As I teased apart tissue with my scalpel during the day, I observed over and over again the difference between the pink, pliable, healthy vessels in the arms and the yellow ones I kept finding around the heart, neck, and legs—slicked with fatty streaks, totally hard, engorged inside with fibrous plaques. I knew I was looking at a riddle. But what was the answer?

In 1984, the team successfully completed the design of the rotary catheter. The Kensey Catheter, as our device came to be called, enabled me to travel around the world, lecturing and visiting hospitals in foreign countries. I was struck by how many physicians were also interested in discovering what really caused atherosclerosis. I was not alone.

But while the device worked beautifully, the atherosclerosis always returned within a few months. Eventually, I made the difficult decision to give up practicing cardiology to devote myself full time to inventing and developing medical devices to help patients.

It was when I was working on a new invention designed to lower blood pressure that I came to understand the significance of the sharp blood-flow peaks so common in elderly people with high blood pressure. No one seemed to have studied this, or the turbulent blood flow that resulted in the arteries. I began working with Dr. Young I. Cho, an engineering professor at Drexel University who had developed computer models of blood flow for NASA and who helped me understand fluid dynamics and shear forces within a closed, pressurized system.

With this new understanding, I was on my way to discovering what I believe is the true cause of atherosclerosis.

It's always sobering when what we've believed were the "facts" about an illness turns out to be wrong. Only twenty years ago, we used to treat gastric ulcers with surgery; today we know that the condition is often caused by a specific bacterium. Ulcers can now be cured with an antibiotic combined with a drug that cuts down stomach acid. In short, new thinking about the origins of an illness helps us better diagnose, measure, and prevent or reverse a disease process.

The pages that follow present some new thinking that logically explains the root cause of atherosclerosis and can help you understand and accurately assess your real risk factors. This theory will help you and your doctor improve the quality of your life and significantly reduce your risk of dying from cardiovascular disease.

We must change our attitude toward atherosclerosis. It *is* preventable, and it may be reversible, if you apply the lifestyle changes recommended in *The Blood Thinner Cure*. Give this book to friends and family, so the people you love can avoid the ravages of this disease. And remember most of all, to teach your children the concepts of a healthy lifestyle.

Kenneth R. Kensey, M.D.

All proceeds I may receive from the sale of this book will go toward further research on the causes and prevention of atherosclerosis.

The Blood Thinner Cure

Part 1

The Basics

I

What Really Causes Atherosclerosis?

Margie is a forty-two-year-old Asian woman, a stockbroker with normal cholesterol, weight, and blood pressure. She never smoked, doesn't exercise, and doesn't have a family history of heart disease and stroke. Ten years ago, she had a hysterectomy, followed by a heart attack four years later. Margie has atherosclerosis.

James is a forty-three-year-old African-American man, a former football player with normal cholesterol and blood pressure. He doesn't smoke, exercises regularly, and has a family history of heart disease and stroke. He began experiencing severe chest pains and headaches during workouts. He carries 275 pounds of solid muscle on his massive frame. James has atherosclerosis.

Michael is a fifty-five-year-old white man, a self-confessed "health nut" and marathon runner, with normal cholesterol, weight, and blood pressure. He has never smoked, eaten a high-fat diet, or been overweight. He does have a family history of heart disease and stroke. Last week, he developed weakness on his left side. Michael has atherosclerosis.

Margie, James, and Michael—all with very different lifestyles and family histories—have few of the traditional risk factors for heart disease and stroke. Yet, each one of them is a heart attack or stroke waiting to happen. What could they all have in common that modern medicine has missed?

They all share a problem, a problem that none of them suspected and that modern medicine has so far almost completely overlooked. Each of them is pumping dangerously thick blood that continuously injures the arteries with each beat. Untreated, this condition will eventually kill them. The problem is that until now, the medical community has looked at their condition as some sort of *biochemical* problem related to high cholesterol, triglycerides, iron, or sugar rather than a *biophysical* problem of pumping thickened blood at abnormally high pressures.

The fact is that one out of every three people in the industrialized world who die this year will succumb to atherosclerosis—a disease characterized by the buildup of bumps of tissue (called plaques) that eventually block stiffened, hardened arteries. If you're like most people, you know very little about the disease that has more than a fifty-fifty chance of ending your life prematurely. What's worse, you're probably not doing the things you need to do *today* to prevent the disease. Unfortunately, many cardiologists still focus on treating atherosclerosis only when it's *too late to reverse the process*. That's partly because up to now, doctors haven't understood what happens in the body that triggers the development of blockages.

There are good reasons why doctors focus on fixing your symptoms instead of preventing artery disease. Blocked arteries are a formidable foe because the problem begins so silently. Until now, the *reason* they form was unknown. Researchers have managed to isolate approximately 300 items that seem to be linked with clogged arteries (including high cholesterol, obesity, smoking, stress, diabetes, lack of exercise, and poor diet), *but none of these things actually triggers the clogging of your arteries.* One-third of the people who do develop atherosclerosis don't have traditional risk factors.

For some reason, Americans seem to accept the idea that hardening of the arteries (arteriosclerosis) and blocked or clogged arteries (atherosclerosis) are tragic but inescapable facts of aging. Most people don't believe for one minute that cancer is inevitable, but we all seem to be strangely resigned to the notion that blocked arteries will one day develop in each one of us if we live long enough.

Atherosclerosis is not inevitable. It's *not* a normal aging process that we just have to accept. The truth is actually quite simple: if you keep your arteries from hardening, you can keep your arteries open forever.

You can prevent heart attacks and strokes.

Not a Chemical Problem

No one has been able to show conclusively why arteries clog only in certain spots and regions in the body. This book uses information from a growing body of research to present the cause of atherosclerosis as mechanical in nature, not biochemical. With this new approach we may be able to explain for the first time the region-specific and site-specific nature of atherosclerosis. Figure 1.1 illustrates the places where atherosclerosis is most likely to occur.

Most doctors will tell you that atherosclerosis is caused by a chemical process: cholesterol and other chemicals in the blood clog the arteries. Yet, even patients with extremely high cholesterol have atherosclerosis in only a few of their arteries. If atherosclerosis were caused *only* by things such as a high-fat diet or high cholesterol, then we would expect to see *all* of the arteries in your body affected—because all of the arteries are exposed to the same blood. But that doesn't happen.

I believe atherosclerosis occurs because your heart has pumped thickened blood at too high a pressure for too long, which *physically* injures certain regions of the arterial system, making the arteries hard and inflexible. Within these hardened regions, blood flow becomes turbulent, and the blood then begins to erode your arteries at specific sites. These sites are often where your arteries branch.

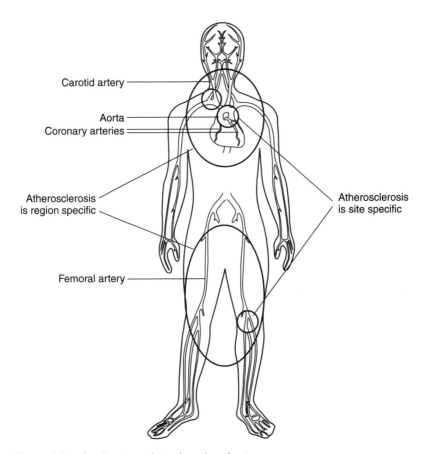

Carotid artery

Aorta
Coronary arteries

Atherosclerosis
is region specific

Atherosclerosis
is site specific

Femoral artery

Figure 1.1   Specific regions and sites where atherosclerosis occurs.

We'll come back to turbulent blood flow and its role in causing arterial injury. For now, keep in mind that if blood flowed through your arteries smoothly (the way water runs through a hose) instead of pulsating with every beat of your heart, you wouldn't get atherosclerosis. You would never get heart disease or stroke.

Why Arteries Harden

For a long time, many scientists thought that hardened arteries and plaques didn't have anything to do with each other—that they occurred independently and that they were perhaps two entirely different processes. I don't agree.

I believe that arteries harden first, and this in turn triggers the formation of blockages—they are directly related. In this book, I'll show that all the risk factors for atherosclerosis have one common denominator: your heart is working too hard because of thickened, sticky blood—what I call "the sludge factor."

When blood is pumped through the flexible arteries of your body, the arteries bulge with each pulsing heartbeat as a way of accommodating the pressure. A child's arteries are very soft and expand effortlessly as the heart pumps, making it easy for the blood to move throughout the body smoothly and quietly. As you age, blood pressure begins to rise, and your blood gets thicker. The blood vessels must cope with higher and higher pressure and thicker and thicker blood. In certain regions this overstretches and injures your arteries. As your blood pressure continues to rise and your blood gets thicker, the heart must work harder to pump the blood. This in turn forces the arteries in the same regions to overstretch even more. This overstretching injures the arteries, which respond to this injury by getting harder to avoid further overstretching.

In recent years, many studies have suggested—and I agree—that atherosclerosis begins with an *injury* to the artery lining that leads to the clogging. What's new is my suggestion that the hardening of the artery wall (arteriosclerosis) is caused by a *physical* injury, not a chemical one. While I believe that diet, lifestyle, and heredity all play a role in mechanically injuring the arteries, the primary cause of artery hardening, as well as the clogging itself, is the way your arteries adapt to this mechanical injury.

Adapt or Die!

If you pumped water through a closed rubber tube at higher and higher pressures, eventually the tube would burst. But your arteries are living tissue, and I believe they have the ability to adapt in response to stress.

As your blood pressure starts to rise, your arteries have a choice: either they adapt to the extra pressure, or they *burst*. An artery adapts by getting tougher and thicker—getting stiffer. In the short run, this saves the arteries from exploding, but as the arteries thicken, they get less flexible, causing the heart to work even harder to pump blood through them.

This adaptation process involves two vicious cycles:

1. As the arteries stiffen, the process triggers higher blood pressure—a never-ending vicious cycle. Figure 1.2 illustrates this cycle. The thickened, hardened arteries (called arteriosclerosis), which occur only in certain regions of the body, cause blood flow to become turbulent within these regions.

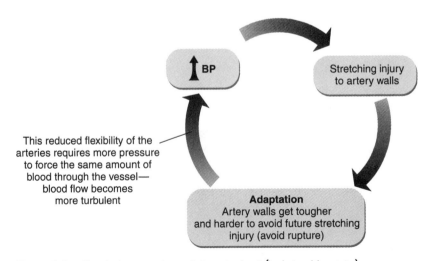

Figure 1.2   The adaptive process that results in arteriosclerosis (hardening of the arteries).

2. Now, in those regions of the body where the arteries have thick-ened and hardened, the turbulent flow begins to "erode" the linings of these arteries at very specific sites, where the arteries branch. Fig-ure 1.3 shows how this occurs. If the erosion were to continue, the artery would eventually wear away, a hole would form, and death would ensue—but that doesn't happen. Instead, the artery protects itself from further erosion by forming a callus (doctors call it plaque). Unfortu-nately, when a callus forms, the "bump" from the callus itself magni-fies the turbulence of the blood flow, causing even more injury, so the callus gets larger. This cycle continues until finally the callus is so big that it stops blood flow altogether, causing a heart attack or stroke.

These two separate processes are part of the continuum of cardio-vascular disease: the arteries first harden and stiffen, which in turn sets off another cycle that ends in blockages.

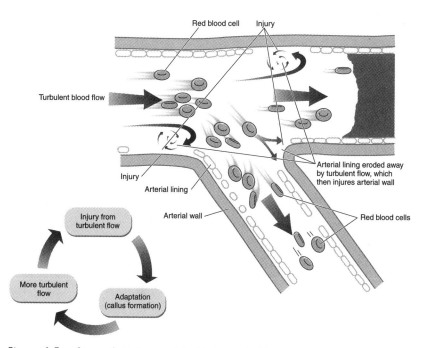

Figure 1.3   Site-specific injuries to arterial wall in a hardened, stiffened artery.

The Overexpansion Zone

When the heart is working overtime to pump blood at higher and higher pressures throughout the body, not all the arteries are exposed to these pressures. So not all become hard and stiff. This has been one of the most puzzling mysteries about the cause of blocked arteries: if diet and lifestyle alone cause artery damage, then why don't the arteries all over the body become stiffened and clogged?

Scientists have long known that blood vessels expand and contract in response to blood flow. What they haven't realized before is the significance of the fact that the arteries closest to the heart and those in the legs are the *first* to become stiff because they are exposed to the most overstretching injury. This constant process of repeated overstretching eventually leads to stiffening and thickening, just as a weight lifter's muscles thicken with the stress of repeated weight lifting.

If you want to find a blocked and clogged artery, the best place to look is in the arteries that feed blood to the heart and brain, what I call the "zone of overexpansion" as shown in Figure 1.4.

Early hardening of the arteries starts in the arteries leading to the heart and brain because these arteries are closest to the heart and are

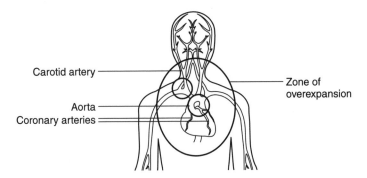

Figure 1.4   Arteries in the zone of overexpansion act like shock absorbers for arteries in the rest of the body.

part of the "zone of overexpansion." As these arteries react to each heartbeat, they get larger and overstretch. They act like shock absorbers for the rest of the arteries in the body. The more the artery overstretches, the more injury to the artery wall, the more it adapts and becomes stiffer and thicker to avoid further injury. Imagine a water balloon: as you fill it, the balloon's walls stretch and stretch. The bigger that water balloon gets, the higher the tension on the walls of the balloon.

Hardened arteries also occur in the legs because when you stand up, gravity drastically boosts the pressure in your legs much more than the pressure in the arteries in other parts of your body. This isn't well known or understood by many doctors, but it's true nevertheless.

The fact that this hardening occurs in these two places first can be understood if you look at the underlying process as a *constant mechanical injury*, not a chemical process such as cholesterol or iron buildup. If hardening of the arteries were a chemical problem, your arteries would harden all over the body—and that just never happens.

As the arteries closest to the heart and in the legs are repeatedly overstretched, they start to stiffen and thicken, especially at the beginning portion of the affected arteries. As explained previously, the thickening response is actually the arteries' way of trying to protect themselves: very forceful blood will overstretch an artery, so it has no choice—it can either rupture, or adapt by thickening and stiffening.

As the arteries stiffen, the blood must be pumped with even more pressure because the resistance to blood flow through a stiffened artery is greater. The left side of the heart pushes harder and faster to try to thrust the blood through the arteries. The blood pressure rises, and the arteries stiffen even more; the more they harden, the higher the blood pressure will rise and the harder the left side of the heart has to work to push blood through the arteries. This is aggravated by stress, coffee, stimulants, and poor diet, which is explained in more detail in later chapters. A vicious, dangerous, and silent cycle begins.

Once the Arteries Harden . . .

Let's review. When you're a child, the blood flows smoothly. Little work is required of the heart to move the blood through soft and supple arteries. But in adulthood, the arteries begin to adapt and then stiffen, which in turn causes the blood flow to become more forceful as it's pumped at higher and higher pressure.

Think of the way a river flows, and you'll have a good picture of the way the blood circulates in your arteries. Is the river clear and fluid, flowing softly and quietly—or a swollen, turgid, raging torrent? Knowing how that river is flowing will help you figure out a lot about the condition of the riverbanks—and knowing how your blood is flowing will reveal how healthy your arteries are. A gently flowing river with lazy currents will have solid banks, but a turgid, boiling torrent will eat away at the river's edge, making the banks crumbly and unstable.

In the same way, if you know how the blood is moving through your vessels (flowing quietly or turbulently) you'll have valuable clues as to the condition of your artery walls.

Of course, it's not quite that simple. A river flows, but your blood pulsates. In fact, the expression "blood flow" is a misnomer: your blood doesn't really "flow" at all. It's forcefully pumped out of the heart and around the body in a pulsating fashion, a continual, unceasing rhythm. As the blood becomes more turbulent and moves back and forth, it swirls around in minipools and eddies, eroding the lining of the arteries. To appreciate the effect, think of the water in your garden hose: if you place a thumb over the nozzle, the spray becomes a blast. It has force, and it has impact.

When the lining of the artery is injured by shear forces caused by the turbulent blood, it begins to protect itself and form a callus, exactly like the callus you'd get on your hands from raking leaves without gloves. As the arteries form these calluses, or plaques, more injury occurs to the vessels: blood moves around the calluses, forming bigger eddies that wear away the sides of the artery even more, like a whirlpool of water eroding the bank of a river. As the callus gets bigger, it creates even more turbulent flow, which leads to more injury and more adaptive response from the arteries.

When Does It Start?

You don't go to bed one night in perfect health and wake up the next day with hardened and clogged arteries. The process of hardening arteries, rising blood pressure, thickening blood, and clogging arteries may begin as early as adolescence. If you really want to stop heart disease, you need to prevent that vicious cycle from ever getting started.

In most people, the whole process begins as blood pressure slowly rises with each decade of life. In some people, that slow rise begins as early as middle childhood. In a few lucky individuals, it never starts at all. There are some eighty-year-olds with very low blood pressure whose arteries will never clog.

Doctors are taught that it's normal for blood pressure to go up as we age, but I don't agree. I believe that as soon as your blood pressure starts to creep up, that signals the onset of the adaptive process—and the result is clogged arteries feeding the heart, brain, or legs.

You and your doctor may be perfectly happy with a blood pressure reading of 110/80—after all, that's not too high—but if last year it was 100/70, your pressure has already started to rise. If your blood pressure is increasing *at all*, even if it's still considered under "normal" limits, the disease process has begun. In another two or three years, your pressure may creep up to 120/85, 130/90, and beyond.

This is significant because we know from the results of the now famous Framingham heart study—which has been following more than 5,000 adults in Framingham, Massachusetts, since 1948 to identify risk factors for heart disease—that people with *very* low blood pressure *never* had heart attacks. If I am right (and this study supports my thinking), there is no such thing as too low a blood pressure (as long as you're not having other symptoms such as weakness or fainting, and you're not going into shock).

Risk Increases as You Age

To prevent arteries from getting blocked, the heart must pump efficiently; it shouldn't have to contract forcefully to move blood out and
around the body. Remember, the harder your heart has to work, the
more abrasive the blood will be as it moves through your arteries. Usually as you age your heart works less efficiently and your blood begins
to be pumped with an ever greater force. The heart then contracts
with incredible ferocity. The arteries must absorb this increasing force
and the result is injury to the artery lining and wall. The older you
get, the more forceful the contraction—and the greater your chance
for a heart attack or stroke.

Atherosclerosis is a disease that dramatically increases after age fifty.
Our shift in thinking from chemical to mechanical explains this age-
related observation.

But this process doesn't happen at the same time to all of us. We
don't all age at the same rate. Do you stay up late, drink lots of alcohol, and eat fat-filled foods? Are you a couch potato who smokes like
an out-of-tune '67 Chevy? If so, odds are your internal organs are aging
a lot faster than those of an athlete who eats lean, healthy foods, gets
plenty of rest, and doesn't smoke.

You may not realize it, but your arteries can age much faster than
the rest of your body, as a result of your genes, lifestyle choices, or
disease. Even youngsters aren't guaranteed healthy arteries if they have
poor health habits. At twenty, you may have the arteries of a fifty-
year-old if you have high blood pressure, diabetes, or kidney disease,
or if you smoke or eat the wrong foods. This is because these diseases
and lifestyle choices force your burdened heart to pump inefficiently,
with much greater force; each time this happens, your arteries are overstretched and injured.

2

High Blood Pressure Will Kill You

We are a nation facing an epidemic of high blood pressure. What we used to call "normal" we now know is too high. The first chapter explained how I believe atherosclerosis begins, rooted in the vicious cycle of high blood pressure, thickened blood, and forceful contraction of the heart. High blood pressure is the one event that triggers the tragic disease of atherosclerosis. That's why we're focusing on it first.

Blood pressure is basically the result of three forces:

- the squeezing of the heart as it pumps blood into the arteries
- the thickness of the blood as it resists blood flow
  (The thickness of the blood is directly related to the work
  the heart is doing.)
- the constriction of smaller arteries

The heart "beat" you can hear through a stethoscope and feel in your pulse is actually the slamming of valves shutting behind the blood to prevent it from flowing back into the heart. Doctors call the contraction of the heart—the *systole* (SIS-tull-ee). The expansion of the heart—the filling phase—is the *diastole* (dy-AS-tull-ee).

When you have your blood pressure taken, the heart's contraction is counted first. The higher (systolic) number represents the pressure while the heart is contracting. The lower (diastolic) number represents the pressure when the heart is filling up with blood between contractions. So, if your blood pressure is 120/80, the "120" represents the force of the contraction, and the "80" is the pressure in the artery while the heart is filling up again.

It appears that blood pressure rates are rising as awareness of the problem falls. As many as 60 million Americans aged six and up have high blood pressure, but 35 percent of them don't realize it. Some experts suspect that this is because we're spending so much time worrying about cholesterol levels that we're ignoring blood pressure. Since high blood pressure usually has no symptoms, many people have high blood pressure for years without knowing it. That's why it's so dangerous.

Anyone can develop high blood pressure, but some people are more likely candidates than others. For example, high blood pressure is more common in blacks than in whites, developing earlier and more severely. In the early and middle adult years, men have high blood pressure more often than women, but the picture changes as men and women age. After menopause, women develop high blood pressure more often than men; about 25 percent of white women and 30 percent of African-American women have high blood pressure—and by age sixty-four, more than half of all women have the problem. Again, most women don't know that they have high blood pressure because at first there are no symptoms. (Once symptoms do appear, they may include headaches, tiredness, dizziness, and shortness of breath, anxiety, or insomnia.)

Finally, heredity can make some families more likely than others to get high blood pressure. If your parents or grandparents had high blood pressure, you may be at higher risk.

High blood pressure doesn't necessarily mean you're tense, nervous, or hyperactive; you can be a calm, relaxed person and still have the problem. Instead, high blood pressure is related to the constriction of the blood vessels and their thickness and flexibility. Also when blood gets thick and sticky, it becomes harder to pump, and more pushing force is required to move it around the body—so, blood pressure rises.

About 90 percent of people with high blood pressure have *essential hypertension,* which means that the precise cause of their blood pressure isn't known; the problem could be linked to genetics, diet, not enough exercise, or obesity. *Secondary hypertension* is far rarer and is caused by a variety of illnesses. In addition, oral contraceptives can raise the blood pressure in some women. Other drugs, such as cocaine or caffeine, may trigger brief minor rises in blood pressure. With further studies, I predict that we will find that most people with essential hypertension have blood that is far too thick and that thinning their blood will reduce their blood pressure.

Diagnosis

The only way you can find out if you have high blood pressure is to have your blood pressure checked often—but it's not really a scientific measure of your health, since your blood pressure changes from moment to moment as you go about your daily life. Taking your blood pressure once a month and saying, "This is my blood pressure," is about as scientifically accurate as measuring a car's speed at any given moment and saying, "This is how fast I always go."

Today's doctors will tell you that blood pressure of less than 120 over 80 is considered ideal for adults, but I believe blood pressure can never be low enough. A systolic pressure (top number) of 130 to 139 or a diastolic pressure (bottom number) of 85 to 89 needs to be watched carefully. Certainly, a blood pressure reading above 140/90 is too high and signals impending danger.

A single elevated blood pressure reading doesn't mean you have high blood pressure, but it's a sign that further observation is required. Ask your doctor how often you should have it checked. Certain problems such as kidney disease can cause high blood pressure, but in 90 to 95 percent of cases, the cause of high blood pressure is unknown.

High pressure readings indicate that the heart is working harder than normal, putting both the heart and the arteries under a greater strain. This contributes to heart attacks, strokes, kidney failure, and a host of other diseases. If high blood pressure isn't treated, the heart may have to work progressively harder to pump enough blood and oxygen to the body's organs and tissues to meet their needs.

What You Can Do

As noted in Chapter 1, high blood pressure leads to more serious health problems. High blood pressure is a life-threatening disease, and you must combat it to avoid the complications of atherosclerosis and stroke. If you've already got high blood pressure, you must get it under control by taking action today. Then you can implement the seven-step plan outlined in Part 2.

Obviously, there are some things you can't do anything about: your age, your family history, your gender, or your race. But many other factors are controllable, including:

- obesity
- alcohol consumption
- fluid consumption
- salt intake
- smoking

- inactivity
- diabetes
- consumption of animal fats

Watch the Weight

A very important tool you have in lowering high blood pressure is to lose weight. As your body weight increases, your blood pressure rises. In fact, being overweight can make you two to six times more likely to develop high blood pressure than if your weight were normal.

Even slight weight loss can make a big difference in helping to prevent high blood pressure. Likewise, if you're obese and you have high blood pressure, losing weight can help lower your pressure.

Most people understand that to lose weight, you need to eat fewer calories than you burn—but don't go on a crash diet to see how quickly you can lose those pounds. It's best to lose weight slowly, about one-half to one pound a week. If you cut back by 500 calories a day by eating less and being more physically active, you can lose about one pound in a week. Losing weight and keeping it off involves a new way of eating and increasing physical activity for life.

The best way to lose weight is to eat a healthy diet in the right amounts (see Chapter 10). By watching out for animal fats and sugar and choosing a diet rich in fruits, vegetables, and low-fat dairy products, you can lower blood pressure dramatically.

Hold the Salt

Some people are more affected by salt than others. Since there's no practical way to predict exactly who will be affected by salt, it makes sense to limit intake to help prevent high blood pressure. A simple rule is not to add salt at the table if you have a problem with high blood pressure.

Exercise

Exercising not only burns calories but also strengthens the heart, releases stress, and can help to lower blood pressure. Regular exercise can be important and helpful, as long as you don't have uncontrolled high blood pressure. However, for people *with* high blood pressure, exercising accelerates the process of arterial injury described in Chapter 1. Therefore, it's imperative that you contact a physician (for a physical examination especially) before starting any sort of exercise program if you know you have a history of high blood pressure.

Change Your Lifestyle

You can lower blood pressure if you make some lifestyle changes. If you smoke, give up the habit. Cutting down on alcoholic drinks and caffeine will also help. Drinking too much alcohol (more than one ounce a day) almost certainly raises blood pressure. And if you're trying to lose weight, remember that alcoholic drinks have calories: about 70–180 per drink, depending on the type. Easing stress is another good way to lower blood pressure (see Chapter 12). Finally, control your blood viscosity and donate blood as often as you can (see Chapter 6). All of these lifestyle changes, if taken together, can be quite effective in lowering blood pressure.

Medication

Changes in eating habits and other lifestyle measures may not lower blood pressure enough; if your doctor has prescribed high blood pressure pills, you must take them as prescribed. These medications will lower your blood pressure and help to keep it under control, which will help prevent strokes and heart attacks and extend the quality and length of your life. Unfortunately, far too many people don't take their medication correctly. You *must* take your medication every day, exactly as your doctor prescribed it, or it just won't work.

If you're having side effects from your medication such as impotence, dizziness, or weight gain, talk to your doctor. There are many drugs from which to choose. It is highly likely that a different drug or combination of drugs will control your blood pressure without untoward symptoms.

Be Obsessive About Blood Pressure

Check your own blood pressure at home on a daily basis. This will give you a good idea of what your blood pressure actually is during your regular daily routine. Measure it at varying times of the day, before and after activities such as walking, eating, gardening, watching television, or playing on the computer. The point is to take your blood pressure at various times of day under different conditions and report it to your physician. Your goal is to have normal blood pressure *all* the time, not just at one time of the day or under certain conditions! Be sure to keep track of the readings in a daily journal.

You can buy a blood pressure monitor kit at most drugstores and through many health catalogs. The arm-cuff products are generally more reliable than the fingertip or wrist models; the automatic inflatable products with digital readout are quick and very convenient, too.

I am currently developing a device that will allow constant measurement of blood pressure without interfering with your daily activities. To treat blood pressure scientifically, we must know what your blood pressure is doing during all daily activities—not just at rest in your doctor's office once a year.

3

The Sludge Factor: The Great Unknown

Mary, forty-five, follows the nurse down the long, antiseptic hallway and sits down quietly in the examination room. With cool, deft fingers, the nurse helps roll up Mary's sleeve and fits a blood pressure cuff on her arm. Stethoscope in her ears, she listens for that first telltale beat of the heart—a healthy 135/80 today. But neither the nurse nor the patient suspects that while Mary's blood pressure seems normal, her blood has thickened dangerously.

The blood pressure monitor doesn't reveal that Mary's blood has turned to sludge, and that the heart's struggle to pump this blood is taking a daily toll on her arteries and her heart.

Just about everybody understands the importance of measuring blood pressure; you can't visit a doctor or hospital without having someone slap an arm cuff on you. But what no one today measures—*although it's every bit as important as blood pressure*—is the thickness of your blood.

You probably don't spend too much time thinking about your blood: how it looks, how it's moving. You may have your blood pressure taken and its components tested, and if the numbers seem normal, you consider yourself healthy and let it go at that. What most people don't understand is that it's not just your blood *pressure* that's important but also its *viscosity*.

What's the Big Deal?

The importance of blood viscosity is quite logical: the easier it is for your heart to pump blood, the healthier your arteries will be—and the healthier your arteries, the healthier your whole body. Blood will be able to reach all the important organs more efficiently. Many factors determine how easily your blood flows through your arteries: how sticky the blood is, how slick it is, how fast it clots, how fast or how gently it flows.

In any complex fluid—whether it's blood, ketchup, or paint—the thinner it is, the less work it takes to pump it. Therefore, the thinner your blood, the easier it is for your heart to pump it around your body, the less the arteries will have to stretch, and the less injury the arteries will sustain. Hurry it along, and it becomes thin and easy to move, like red wine; leave it to pool and puddle, and it becomes thick, muddy, and sludgy, driven to clot.

Your blood is a combination of red and white blood cells, plasma, lipids, proteins, and platelets—a complex slurry that gets thinner depending on how fast it flows. But many other things affect how thick or thin your blood is (for example, high blood pressure, smoking, male gender, elevated cholesterol, obesity, diabetes, dehydration, and infection). Unfortunately, there is no organ in the body that monitors the viscosity of blood. The kidneys make sure the blood has the right concentration of critical components, but they can't directly check viscosity.

Think of the blood as a liquid organ that feeds all the other organs and eliminates their garbage. If it isn't working well, the rest of the organs will get sick. In fact, each cell in your body depends on blood for oxygen and nutrients. The lower the viscosity, the healthier all your cells will be.

Red Blood Cell Concentration

The most important factor in determining blood thickness is how *many* red blood cells you have (in other words, their *concentration*). Blood is almost 50 percent red blood cells, although the actual concentration (called the *hematocrit*) varies from one person to the next.

Men have a naturally higher amount of red blood cells (the normal hematocrit range for men is between 37 percent and 49 percent; for premenopausal women, it's between 34 percent and 46 percent). The higher the concentration of red blood cells, the harder your heart must work to pump the blood. A 10 percent increase in your hematocrit means a 25 percent increase in your blood's thickness. This is one reason why men are more prone to heart attacks than premenopausal women.

Both in the operating room and in the morgue, I was regularly amazed by the fact that some people's blood was so thick and sticky that it was almost impossible to get the blood off of my surgical gloves after I had finished an operation or an autopsy. You could see the difference when you poured a test tube full of blood into a sink; some washed easily down the drain, but other blood clung to the sides and left a dark, stubborn stain behind in the sink. If your blood is thick and sticky because of a high concentration of red blood cells, your heart is pumping sludge.

Red Blood Cell Flexibility

The second most important factor that determines blood thickness is how flexible your red blood cells are. Because red blood cells are almost three times as big as the capillaries through which they travel, they must be flexible in order to move easily throughout the body. Because of their shape-shifting ability, healthy red blood cells bend and curve and bounce like an animated cartoon character as they navigate the twists and turns of the arteries. These doughnut-shaped cells must flex if they want to squeeze through capillaries one-third their size. In fact, if red blood cells *weren't* able to bend and squeeze, blood would be a solid, not a liquid. This is why the more flexible your red blood cells, the easier your blood will flow and the thinner your blood will be.

The flexibility of a red blood cell is most affected by two variables:

- the age of the cell
- what is dissolved in the surrounding plasma

One of the reasons why premenopausal women have such a low incidence of atherosclerosis is that they lose blood each month, which triggers the production of new, flexible young red blood cells. Once women reach menopause and their monthly supply of flexible blood cells decreases, they become equally vulnerable to heart attacks. If men could simulate menstruation, I believe they too would almost eliminate early-age heart attacks and stroke.

Basically, the younger your red blood cells, the more flexible they are. When these cells are young, they bend and stretch and willingly change shape, helping the blood ooze easily around the curves of the arteries and through the capillaries.

But since red blood cells live for only about 120 days, it doesn't take long before they start to become less flexible. Eventually, they adapt to being oversqueezed. They become tough and rigid. At the end of their life span, these cells have adapted by transforming from soft, mushy grapes to tough, inflexible raisins. After 120 days, these old red blood cells are removed by the spleen.

In people with diabetes, these inflexible red blood cells are pushed through capillaries, scouring the lining of the capillaries much like the work of a Brillo pad. The arteries adapt to the injury by closing themselves off. Blindness all too often results from the movement of these inflexible red blood cells through the tiniest of the capillaries in the eyes. It's also the reason people with diabetes lose kidneys and legs—the capillaries are shutting off because of inflexible blood cells.

Plasma Thickness

The thickness of your blood is also determined by the thickness of the plasma that surrounds the blood cells, which can turn to sludge in the presence of chronic infections and inflammations.

Where there is inflammation in the body (from artery damage itself, long-term inflammation, or infection from any cause), the blood becomes thicker and stickier. It would seem especially prudent, then, for people with frequent or chronic bacterial or viral infections (or chronic inflammatory diseases such as arthritis, allergies, asthma, or lupus) to pay particular attention to their blood viscosity and try to keep it low by the methods we describe in this book.

Cholesterol

Doctors focus on lowering cholesterol to reduce the risk of atherosclerosis, and for good reason: it works—but not the way everyone thinks. Cholesterol doesn't cause atherosclerosis, but it does increase viscosity, which in turn injures the lining of arteries. This may sound heretical.

Long ago, when the hot air balloon was first invented, Ben Franklin himself thought that the balloon rose because of the smoke billowing into it—not realizing that it wasn't the smoke, but the hot air, that made the balloon rise. People could *see* the smoke as the balloon rose, but they never noticed that the true cause of the balloon's rising was the hot air. They had no way to measure the temperature accurately.

It's the same with cholesterol and blood viscosity. Cholesterol is a lot easier to measure than blood viscosity. Cholesterol levels have been measured for decades, and high levels of cholesterol do elevate your risk for heart attacks and stroke—not because of the cholesterol itself, but because the cholesterol increases the thickness of your blood.

In this book, I refer to cholesterol and other fats as simply "blood fat." In my view, animal fats are large, globular molecules that make blood thicker; those same fat molecules are naturally made in massive amounts by the body and are necessary for normal function. But when there is too much fat in the blood, these molecules thicken the blood.

Other Influences

Cigarette smoking, high levels of blood fats, diabetes, elevated homo-cysteine (an amino acid), and a wide range of other health conditions also increase blood thickness and stickiness. In addition, many diseases increase blood thickness by making red blood cells less flexible (as in dia-betes or kidney disease) or by increasing their concentration (as in sleep apnea).

Genetic Link

Extremely thick blood may also be genetic. Many different groups of people are genetically predisposed to high blood fats (cholesterol and triglycerides). These people have a much higher incidence of athero-sclerosis because they have a very high blood viscosity. Most must take drugs to lower their cholesterol. Elevated viscosity may be the reason why so many people have a family history of heart disease and strokes of "unknown cause" or with no other well-accepted risk factors.

The Role of Inflammation and C-Reactive Protein (CRP)

As atherosclerosis develops, the injured arteries become inflamed, which increases blood viscosity. As the artery's lining is injured, it releases C-reactive protein (CRP) into the bloodstream. Measuring this protein's level indicates how much injury is occurring to the artery's lining. I believe CRP is a marker for a person's risk of heart attack or stroke. Figure 3.1 demonstrates this inflammation cycle.

Researchers knew that the higher the concentration of CRP, the more likely a man was to have a heart attack or stroke. Now scientists at Brigham and Women's Hospital and Harvard Medical School have found that high CRP levels also predict future heart disease among

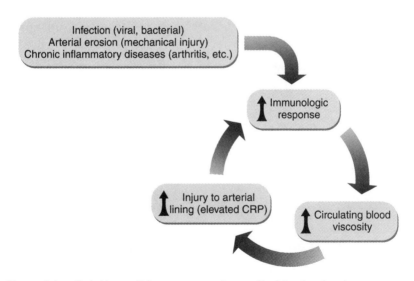

Figure 3.1   The body's natural inflammatory response increases blood viscosity and accelerates atherosclerosis.

healthy women. In fact, women with the highest levels of CRP were five times more likely than those with the lowest levels to suffer from any heart problem, and seven times more likely to have a heart attack or stroke, according to the March, 23, 2000 issue of the *New England Journal of Medicine.* The high protein levels were able to accurately predict future heart problems even among otherwise low-risk women such as nonsmokers, women with normal cholesterol, women with no family history of heart disease, women without diabetes, and women with normal blood pressure.

These findings indicate that measuring CRP may presently be one of the most accurate ways to screen for the risk of heart attack or stroke because blood levels of this protein in at-risk people begin to rise six to eight years before a first heart attack or stroke. A high CRP level is probably a warning that your blood is too thick, your blood pressure is too high, or a combination of both—and that it's time to put my seven-step blood thinning program to work.

No one knows for certain what causes this low-grade inflammation that seems to put otherwise healthy people at risk, but researchers suggest that an infection may contribute to the artery-damaging process. Possible infectious triggers include bacteria such as *Chlamydia pneumoniae* and *Heliocobacter pylori,* and viral agents such as herpes simplex virus and cytomegalovirus. It could be that antibiotics or antiviral agents will someday help to prevent artery damage.

Measuring Blood Viscosity

Until recently, many scientists didn't realize how important the viscosity (let alone other biophysical parameters) of your blood can be to your overall health—especially the health of your arteries—in part because there was no practical way to measure it accurately and in a useful way.

The idea that the viscosity of your blood could be an important cause of artery disease may seem almost heretical today—new ideas often are. Just a few years ago, doctors who said that a common bacterium caused most cases of ulcers and could be cured by antibiotics would have been laughed out of the hospital. But today, we know it's true. For most people—including many doctors—the idea of measuring blood thickness is just as foreign a concept today as measuring blood pressure was 200 years ago.

In the early 1700s, doctors had no idea how to measure blood pressure, or even that it was an important indicator of heart health. We didn't even know that blood pressure *existed* until clergyman Stephen Hales first measured it in 1731. It would be another 170 years before Harvey Cushing finally introduced an Italian version of the modern blood pressure cuff to the United States and persuaded American doctors to use the newfangled device.

Just as doctors had no idea how to measure blood pressure in the 1700s, that's pretty much where we are today with the measurement of blood viscosity. We *know* that thickened, sticky blood is not healthy; after more than thirty years of study using primitive measurement methods, an ever-growing group of scientists realizes that thick, sludgy blood is linked to artery disease. But how dangerous is thickened blood, and why must we strive so desperately to get this "sludge factor" under control?

Ten years ago, when Drexel University research scientist Dr. Young Cho and I worked with a computer simulation of blood flow developed for NASA, we realized how important blood thickness is. Once we ascertained that certain types of blood flow can injure arteries at the same sites where plaques form in atherosclerosis, we wanted to measure viscosity—but there wasn't a simple, reliable device to do it. It took us ten years to develop a bedside instrument sensitive, simple, quick, and accurate enough to effectively measure a person's blood thickness, a device now in clinical trials around the country.

Once doctors begin measuring blood thickness as often as they measure blood pressure, more people will begin to understand its importance. Until we do that, we are missing one of the three big factors that affect the work of the heart—and the energy that our arteries are absorbing moment by moment, day by day.

I predict that being able to accurately measure the factors that make blood flow will be as important to understanding diseases of the arteries as the discovery of the light microscope was to the treatment of bacterial diseases. Until Robert Koch discovered the anthrax bacillus in 1876 with his light microscope, scientists were unaware of the role that bacteria play in human disease. Likewise, without an accurate viscometer, scientists have not been able to understand the role that blood thickness plays in artery disease, asthma, and arthritis.

In the next five years, as these devices to measure blood viscosity are made available, I predict that everyone will realize how important blood viscosity and other factors (like stickiness, slickness, and abrasiveness) that affect blood flow can be—just as the realization of the importance of the light microscope revolutionized the treatment of bacterial disease 125 years ago.

4

I Am Harry's Artery

Like many Midwesterners of a certain age, Harry D.* kept his feelings mostly to himself. His life had not been easy, and its vicissitudes were more extreme than most. But it was Harry's arteries that bore the brunt of his lifestyle.

Although Harry's parents were poor and farm life was hard, there was a ready supply of cream, butter, lard-crust pies, and meat canned with hot fat.

I am Harry's aorta. I carry the blood from his heart in a smooth and silken flow, gently moving whisper-soft throughout his body. I am young and flexible, and the movement is effortless.

As a child, Harry was exposed to both his mother's overeating and secondhand smoke from his father's cigarettes. Eggs and porridge with thick cream were the only ways to greet the day, followed by a large lunch and dinner, both with dessert. No holiday, birthday, special

---

*We've taken literary license in this chapter; Harry D. is a composite of several patients I have treated.

event, or achievement on Harry's part went by without a homemade pie or cake in celebration. At the same time, whenever Harry's father was in the house, a pale gray nimbus of cigarette smoke encircled everyone's head.

I am Harry's aorta. I carry along the blood from the heart. The blood is getting thicker and heavier; his heart must squeeze harder to push it out and up into me. These spurts of blood are hard and rough, and my sides bulge out in response to each beat. Still, I am young, and all things are possible.

Atherosclerosis caught up with Harry's father when Harry was ten; a fatal heart attack dropped the fifty-four-year-old farmer like a stone as he was sweating in the hot sun, out in the cornfield under a perfectly blue August sky. He fell without sound or preamble; the cornstalks largely cushioned his fall. After that, Harry had to take care of the twins, as well as his mother, as best he could in the mornings and evenings after school and his farm work.

In high school, when his siblings were old enough to share the work, Harry began a serious program of weight lifting designed to increase his strength and bulk. Each day after school before running home to farm chores, the gangly teenager escaped to the gym, where he lifted increasingly heavy weights—sweating, grunting, and holding his breath until the veins all over his body seemed ready to pop out of his skin. He reckoned that bulking up would make him more manly. But Harry's mother wouldn't have allowed this activity had she realized that each hoist of a 300-pound barbell caused Harry's blood pressure to soar from his normal reading of 90/60 to 350/200.

I am Harry's aorta. There are explosions in the blood. When each explosion comes, the blood is like nothing I have ever known. Harder, faster, rougher, each spurt moving up is like a collision, and I'm afraid I'll burst. Each pulse makes me wonder how I will recover. I must put down a new layer of cells to protect myself. I must get tougher.

In 1940, Harry—now eighteen—joined the army. The stress of worrying about the farm and how his family would manage without him made the transition even harder than it might have been under ordinary circumstances. But these weren't ordinary circumstances; the country was at war. The homesick private went through pack after pack of Chesterfields, and his blood pressure was now 115/75—well within "normal" limits but a dramatic increase from his previous level of 90/60. About this same time, Harry became a social drinker, and the increased level of alcohol in his body only added to his dehydration.

I am the femoral artery feeding blood to Harry's leg. With each step, the blood is heavy, pushing down along my length. I am pushed out farther than I should have to go. There is no escape from the pushing, pounding blood. I'm afraid of bursting. I must lay down more cells for protection: I must stiffen. I will stiffen most at places where I can't escape from the blood's rough punches.

I am the aorta. The blood is heavy, thick and very sticky, so much tougher to move. It pulls at the branches of the smaller arteries. The heart hammers with each pulse. This blood is turbulent; it swirls and eddies, moving up into my arch and into my branches. It tears at patches of my lining, inflaming and trying to wear a hole in me. It flows around corners with such force, dragging back and forth across my lining like sandpaper. Where the tearing and dragging are worst, where I have been stretched the most, where I am stiffest, I have wounded streaks like shiny scars. I must build up extra cells on my lining to protect from further erosion. But the more I build up, the more the blood is agitated. Yet, I have no choice.

In 1942, Harry was captured by the Japanese and imprisoned in a concentration camp. Stripped of privileges (no cigarettes) and starved, he survived mostly on thin gruel, pieces of bread, and an occasional root vegetable that he secretly scavenged while working the fields. Because of the monsoon season, there was always plenty of water to drink in the camp. After eight months, Harry had lost 90 pounds and his blood pressure had fallen to 100/60. At this point, the cycle of artery injury began to reverse itself as Harry's body ate up all its fats and any extra tissue in an attempt to survive.

> *The blood is quiet now and gentle, like an old friend. It's even thinner and calmer than the blood I knew when I was young, and no longer sticky. The heart is quieter, too; it takes so little to move this fine and gentle blood, gliding smoothly around my branches. It doesn't stick or tear. I feel my cellular defenses dissolving and my stiffness beginning to relax. I am letting go. I am becoming soft and supple once again. I welcome the incoming blood with my new elasticity.*

Harry came home in 1944, married his high school sweetheart, and went to night school on the GI bill. He also started smoking again and eating fatty foods, and he gained back his lost weight (and then some). Although he didn't realize it, he began to develop diabetes. He became more and more stressed as he struggled to get his degree and support a family, which now included a baby, Harry Jr. There was no time for relaxation or exercise, and his blood pressure crept up to 120/80.

> *I am the aorta. Once more, the blood has become heavy, thick, and forceful. Now each pulse is punishing, hard-edged, pushing out my sides too far, too fast. I am losing my recoil. I am struggling to recover. I must not rip apart, and so I thicken. I thicken.*

> *I am a red blood cell. As I flow through the river of plasma, the water is pulled out of me. I begin to shrink, wrinkle, and become stiff. I no longer slide easily through the little capillaries.*

By 1950, through perseverance and drive, Harry had managed to work himself up to vice president of an architectural firm. He never minded the long hours, most of them spent standing over a drafting table. His type A personality seemed to thrive on stress, and the constant cigarettes and countless cups of coffee a day kept him perpetually keyed up. His wife hoped that with a new promotion, Harry might slow down and take better care of himself—but Harry didn't have time for that. His blood pressure was now 130/85, his weight had peaked at 230, and his sugar level was getting higher.

I am the coronary artery. I have become thick and tough now. I feel the turbulence of the roiling blood; by the time it reaches me, it's so much thicker that I can barely stand its wearing, sticky erosion. I start to form calluses at my branches. I thicken more in order to survive. I thicken.

I am a capillary. The stiff red blood cells have begun to scour my lining, so I am thickening to protect myself.

Over the next ten years, Harry began his own successful business, only to lose it by going bankrupt. His children thought the business failure was related to his wife's death from heart disease in late 1959. By 1960, devastated by his wife's death and the failure of his business, Harry had developed a severe bleeding ulcer and was drinking heavily. Although he took antacids, the ulcer wasn't healing, and each day he would lose some blood. Harry was too depressed to eat, and he lost fifty pounds during the first six months of the year. His blood pressure went back down to 120/80.

I am the aorta. The blood is easier now, lighter and thinner. Its pulse is kinder, not something to fear. The heart is squeezing much more gently. There is calm now. I am easing. I am shedding my defenses. Once more, I am becoming alive, elastic; I can easily carry the blood.

By 1968, Harry had got his life back on track. He had stopped smoking and drinking and had remarried. Unfortunately, he regained all the weight he had lost and more. (His new wife was not only a gourmet cook but also part owner of a restaurant.) Harry's weight now ballooned to 250 pounds, and he was finally diagnosed as a diabetic. His doctor gave him medicine for controlling his sugar and told him that he must lose weight.

But Harry was back on the career treadmill, working his way up in a new firm; within seven years, he once more became a vice president. Once again, his work and his life had no room for healthy foods or exercise, and he continued to struggle with his weight and his diabetes, which was often out of control.

> *I am the capillary, living on the fringes in the eyes, the legs, and the kidneys. The red blood cells will no longer bend as they travel through me. They are hard and wounding, each one too big, too wide, slicing and tearing along my whole length. They tear my lining and wear it away; I thicken to survive. The red blood cells will soon no longer pass my way.*

By 1975, Harry was diagnosed with soaring cholesterol and triglyceride levels well above 300, and his diabetes was uncontrolled. He started getting insulin injections, and because his blood pressure had climbed to 150/100, he was put on a diuretic, which removed water from blood, increasing his blood thickness—as did the diabetes and the fats in his blood. Ironically, the insulin injections seemed to increase his appetite, which made his struggle with weight even harder, and his lifelong preference for high-fat foods certainly didn't help the situation.

> *I am the aorta. I am rigid and unbending. The blood flow stops between each heartbeat, then is sent flying, tearing and pulling at my lining. Now there is no going back. This blood is thicker than ever and sometimes so sticky, filled with fatty debris. Where I am most inflamed, I am building up calluses. I am the aorta; I am the artery feeding the brain, the heart, and the legs.*

Harry was about to celebrate his fifty-eighth birthday when, in the first days of November 1980, he began to feel severe chest pains. His company sent him to the Cleveland Clinic, where his blood pressure was recorded at 160/100 and an angiogram revealed that his coronary arteries were almost completely closed. A triple bypass followed; it took Harry almost a year to fully recover from it.

Five years later, Harry began experiencing severe leg cramps and numbness in his feet, as his diabetes triggered the artery thickening process to continue into the smallest arteries in his legs and feet. Because of his uncontrolled diabetes, his red blood cells were no longer flexible, and they couldn't move through the capillaries without causing damage, so the capillaries began to close off. Since the smallest capillaries are in the feet, eyes, and kidneys, this is where capillary damage first became obvious in Harry's case. Soon Harry had cramps in his right leg that were so severe that he couldn't walk more than 100 yards down the street before the pain forced him to sit down. His doctor found that his diabetes was out of control, and he started taking a higher dose of insulin. An angiogram of the leg showed a blocked artery that appeared to be partly calcified; he was sent for a balloon angioplasty.

I am the femoral artery. The blood can no longer move through me; all along my length I have built up thick, hardened calluses. My thickened places are hardening and dying, and I am dying. Dying all along my length.

The angioplasty was successful, and Harry was once again able to walk normally. But something had changed Harry's spirit; he could no longer summon the drive that had fueled his career successes. With his wife's encouragement, he made the difficult decision to retire. Harry and his wife bought a farm in Wisconsin. His oldest son, fearful about his parents' ability to manage alone, also moved there with his family.

On a dark morning in February 1987, as Harry chipped ice from the animals' feeding trough, he felt the cramps return to his right leg, and he realized at the same moment that the ones in his left leg had now become much worse. This time, the angiogram showed that the arteries below the knees in both legs were seriously blocked. Harry was sent for bypass grafts in both legs.

I am the artery below the knee; I am thick and tough, and hardly any blood can pass through me.

I am the femoral artery, and I am concrete, filled with rotting, rusty debris, a bent and twisted thing.

I am the aorta. I am thick and hard, gnarled and snakelike.

The bypass grafts bought Harry some time. Unfortunately, they were doing nothing to stop the deadly end-stage disease from progressing elsewhere in his body. In fact, because of his diabetes, even the leg bypass grafts clotted off; the capillary damage was too severe. By 1989, he was showing signs of kidney and eye problems as well as the loss of feeling in the feet. His blood pressure had gone up to 180/110. After he switched to the newest type of blood pressure medication, his blood pressure dropped to 150/95. But Harry wasn't good at remembering to take his medication. The disease progressed. The toes on Harry's foot turned black, the skin on his right leg an awful contrast in deathly white. There was no pulse around the ankles; his right leg had to be amputated.

Harry's wife said later that when Harry lost his leg, she lost Harry. No longer able to walk, he became depressed, angry, and extremely hard to get along with. His personality seemed to have been permanently changed; the person who now inhabited Harry's body bore little resemblance to the man she had married. In 1991, his first heart attack killed a third of his heart muscle. He was rushed into surgery and given a second three-way bypass. Harry survived the surgery, although he no longer cared. He began to smoke again. In 1992, he experienced a classic "ministroke."

I am the carotid artery, and I feed the brain. How the blood must stagger to get past my hardened defenses; large mountains of tissue grow from my walls. The blood flow is turbulent and harsh, pulling on me as it passes by. It falters, pools, and clots; it picks up debris from my plaques. I narrow further, closing off.

Harry was scheduled for an operation to remove the blocked part of his carotid artery, although the anesthesiologist considered him extremely high risk because of his weight, his diabetes, and his previous surgeries. No one gave Harry very good odds, and yet, there seemed to be no choice.

Unfortunately, Harry did not survive. During the surgery, Harry suffered a fatal heart attack. He died three days before his seventieth birthday in November 1992.

5

Tune-Up in the Body Shop

Jane and Sam each bought a brand-new sporty American car ten years ago. Jane was a sensible driver who never missed a tune-up. Every 5,000 miles, she changed her oil, and she diligently followed the recommendations for changing points and plugs. At 200,000 miles, her car was still humming. Sam, on the other hand, was an auto cowboy who slipped, rode, and popped his clutch and regularly drove over almost impossible terrain. When he finally got around to a tune-up, the oil was so thick and sludgy that it looked more like molasses than motor oil. Kept outside in all weather and never washed or waxed, by 100,000 miles, his car was ready for the junkyard.

You know that if your car is going to last, you've got to change the oil, wash off corrosive salts and road debris, balance the tires, adjust the alignment, flush out the radiator, use the right gas, and tune up the engine. You wouldn't expect a car to last if it hasn't been treated to a regular inspection and maintenance schedule—especially if you drive it hard for a long time. Yet, many people ask their arteries to put up with very much the same sort of abuse.

Most people would never treat their cars the way Sam treated his—but how many of us take the time to do a little preventive maintenance on our bodies? Do you get physicals on a regular basis? Have you ever heard of your homocysteine, much less had it tested? Have you taken a stress test before starting a running program or had a baseline echocardiogram?

It's time for a tune-up in the body shop.

Prevention Is the Key

Preventing atherosclerosis—like preventing cancer—is important because once atherosclerosis develops, there's a point beyond which you can't stop the spread of the disease. Right now, we don't know exactly where that point is—so, prevention is what you've got to aim for. Prevention is also important because bypass surgery and balloon angioplasty are mere Band-Aids that do nothing to stop the disease.

So, how do you do that? By getting a physical and taking a number of tests to find out how healthy you are right now—and by following my seven-step plan presented here to stop atherosclerosis, which will in turn lower blood pressure, decrease the force of the heart's contraction, and lower blood viscosity. But it's a plan you must follow for life if you want to avoid the ravages of atherosclerosis.

Simple Seven-Step Plan

The most important way to stop atherosclerosis is to keep your blood pressure low and keep your blood thin. **Once your blood pressure is under control**, follow this seven-step plan, and your blood will stay thin and slick:

1. Donate blood regularly to help keep it thin.
2. Lubricate your blood: take a low-dose aspirin tablet, a fish oil capsule, and vitamins daily.

3. Try to stop smoking.
4. Try to drink ten to twelve glasses of water daily.
5. Eat a diet low in animal fat and stimulants.
6. Get plenty of the right kind of exercise.
7. Ease stress in your life.

Get a Physical

First and foremost, before you begin this or any other health or exercise program, you should have a complete physical at your family doctor's office to check out your general health. Be sure the physical includes a blood pressure check (during exercise, if possible).

Help Your Doctor Help You

Patients must learn how to speak up and ask for the care they need, especially when it comes to atherosclerosis.

Before your appointment:

- Write down your concerns.
- Keep a diary of symptoms so that you can describe them clearly.
- Write down any past treatments.
- Be sure to have any drugs you're taking with you at the appointment.
- Write down your family medical history.
- Ask a friend or relative whom you trust to accompany you to help listen and understand.

During the office visit:

- Be open and honest, especially about alcohol or drug abuse.
- Describe your symptoms: when they started, how often they occur, and if they've been getting worse.

- Note any stress in your life.
- Ask questions, and ask for supporting literature or videos.
- Be sure you understand what the health care provider says; ask for an explanation of any unfamiliar terms.
- If your doctor prescribes medication, make sure you understand the instructions (when to take it, what to do if you forget, what foods or drugs to avoid while taking it, what side effects may occur, and so forth).
- Take notes.

Blood Tests

Get them all! Blood tests are relatively inexpensive and can detect a number of asymptomatic but devastating diseases. A number of blood tests are often part of a physical, but if your doctor doesn't order them automatically, you'll need to ask him or her to do so (all routinely available):

- hematocrit (concentration of red blood cells)
- blood fats and total cholesterol with HDL and LDL breakdown
- triglycerides
- homocysteine

Hematocrit

Your hematocrit is the measure of the concentration of red blood cells. As your hematocrit increases, blood viscosity rises exponentially: a 10 percent increase in your hematocrit will mean a 25 percent increase in your blood thickness. The value currently considered to be "normal" is between 35 percent and 45 percent (it will vary depending on your sex and age); ideally, it should be between 35 percent and 40 percent.

The test itself is reliable and inexpensive (about $4) and takes only five to ten minutes. At present, there is no self-test for hematocrit levels. You can have the test performed at a commercial lab, a hospital, or your doctor's office, and you don't need to avoid eating or drinking beforehand. The test requires only a few minutes in the laboratory, but it may take anywhere from a few minutes to a few days before the results are reported to your doctor.

Blood Fats and Cholesterol

There are two major categories of cholesterol that you need to understand: the "good" cholesterol (high-density lipoprotein, or *HDL cholesterol*) and the "bad" cholesterol (low-density lipoprotein, or *LDL cholesterol*).

LDL cholesterol and triglycerides are large molecules of fatlike globules carried in your blood. Too much LDL cholesterol dramatically increases viscosity (probably by causing your red blood cells to clump together). A high level of LDL cholesterol in the blood is a primary risk factor for atherosclerosis because it is essentially a simple way of measuring viscosity. Some studies show that there is no such thing as too low an LDL level when it comes to decreasing atherosclerosis. In fact, there is a direct relationship between levels of LDL cholesterol and heart disease.

Your body makes most of the LDL cholesterol you have, while the rest comes from animal products that you eat, such as red meats, eggs, butter, cheese, and whole milk. We need some fats in the blood to form cell membranes, brain cells, some hormones, and other tissues, and to help the body synthesize bile acids and vitamin E. I suspect that the body can make as much cholesterol as it needs to function normally. Additional cholesterol from animal fats will certainly not *thin* your blood.

On the other hand, your body makes HDL cholesterol for your protection. I believe it acts like a lubricant—like oil in your car, allowing

IF YOU WANT TO LOWER BLOOD FAT . . .

In order to lower blood fat content, there are several things you can do:

- Try to lose weight: even a small weight loss helps lower blood fats.
- Start to exercise: aerobic exercise several times a week can lower blood fats.
- Cut down on smoking: our early studies suggest that smoking makes blood stickier. If you can't stop, try to cut down.

blood to flow through the arteries without causing damage. HDL cholesterol may even lay down a film on the lining of the artery wall to protect it. HDL is made up of very small molecules—the opposite of LDL. Think of them as little ball bearings that help move the blood along.

Until blood viscosity is routinely measured, knowing your total blood cholesterol level is an important first step in determining your risk for heart disease, but don't stop there. While a total cholesterol count is helpful, you'll also want to break it down into LDL and HDL cholesterol. Ideally, what you want is a high level of HDL and a low level of LDL. If your doctor orders only a total cholesterol count, insist on a breakdown of LDL and HDL. Remember: *LDL cholesterol is a better predictor of heart attack risk than total blood cholesterol, and LDL is proportionate to the thickness of blood.*

It's worth getting a full lipid profile after a twelve-hour overnight fast in order to determine your triglycerides, HDL, and LDL, and then talk with your doctor about the results. Look at the HDL as an indication of how much "lubricant" you have in your arteries. It's also possible to have a reasonable LDL and a low HDL, which isn't good. What

CHOLESTEROL LEVELS

Total Cholesterol

Less than 200 mg/dL	Desirable
200 to 239 mg/dL	Borderline
240 mg/dL and above	High

Children Ages 2–19

Less than 170 mg/dL	Acceptable
170 to 199 mg/dL	Borderline
200 mg/dL and above	High

HDL Cholesterol

Less than 35 mg/dL	Low
40 to 50 mg/dL (male)	Average
50 to 60 mg/dL (female)	Average

LDL Cholesterol

Less than 130 mg/dL	Desirable
130 to 159 mg/dL	Borderline
160 mg/dL and above	High

Children Ages 2–19

Less than 110 mg/dL	Acceptable
110 to 129 mg/dL	Borderline
130 mg/dL and above	High

mg/dL = milligrams per deciliter

you want to see is a high level of HDL and a low level of LDL. Check the chart above for desirable rates.

Keep in mind that you may have normal LDL, HDL, and total cholesterol counts and still have very thick, highly viscous blood for some other reason. *Cholesterol is only part of the story.* In one new study reported in the March 2000 issue of the journal *Atherosclerosis,* cholesterol levels were found to be under the "danger" level for 750 men and women who were diagnosed with serious blockages of their coronary arteries. In fact, in this study, 51 percent of the men who needed a heart bypass had cholesterol levels below 200 mg/dL.

Triglycerides

Triglycerides are the chemical form in which most fat exists in food and in your blood. You produce triglycerides from fats you eat or that your body makes from other energy sources, such as carbohydrates. The calories from your food that aren't used right away by your body tissues are converted to triglycerides and stored in fat cells. When you need energy, your hormones trigger the release of triglycerides from fat tissue.

A high level of triglycerides in your blood, like cholesterol, is linked to coronary artery disease, and for the same reasons. A high triglyceride level means your blood will be very thick. Triglyceride levels are measured by a blood test taken after an overnight food, beverage, and alcohol fast.

TRIGLYCERIDE LEVELS

Less than 200 mg/dL	Normal
200 to 400 mg/dL	Borderline–high
400 to 1,000 mg/dL	High
Above 1,000 mg/dL	Very high

mg/dL = milligrams per deciliter

Note: The normal triglyceride values are age related; while there is some controversy over the most appropriate normal ranges, the younger you are, the lower your normal rate should be. From birth to age twenty-nine, a normal reading is below 140; from ages thirty to thirty-nine, below 150; from ages forty to forty-nine, below 160; and from ages fifty to fifty-nine, below 200. In my opinion, there is no such thing as too low a level of triglycerides or too low an LDL level; the lower they are, the thinner your blood.

Homocysteine

Homocysteine is an amino acid (a building block of protein) that has been linked to a higher risk of coronary artery disease and stroke, even among people with normal cholesterol levels. I believe that abnormal homocysteine levels may contribute to hardening of the arteries by decreasing red blood cell flexibility, thus again increasing blood thickness. Recent studies suggest that elevated blood homocysteine levels are as important as high blood fat levels as a risk factor for atherosclerosis.

In one recent study, researchers found a direct relationship between homocysteine levels and severity of artery blockages. For every 10 percent rise in homocysteine, there was nearly the same rise in the risk of developing severe coronary heart disease. Another recent study has found that postmenopausal women with higher homocysteine levels also had a higher rate of coronary heart disease. Between 10 percent and 20 percent of coronary heart disease cases have been linked to high homocysteine levels.

High levels may be caused by hereditary or dietary factors. Some people have high levels of homocysteine because they have inherited a defective gene from both parents. (If you get the defective gene from only one parent, you may have a slightly high homocysteine level.) About one out of every 100 people carries one such gene.

It's also possible to have a high homocysteine level if you don't get enough folic acid, vitamin B_6, or vitamin B_{12} in your diet. Supplementation with one or more of these vitamins can lower your homocysteine level *no matter what the cause, and it costs next to nothing.*

Homocysteine is measured by a simple blood test taken at any time of the day. You don't need to stop eating or drinking before the test. Most hospital labs can measure homocysteine, or a blood sample can be sent out to a special laboratory.

The laboratory test can be obtained for about $40.

HOMOCYSTEINE LEVELS

Between 5 and 15 μmol/L	Normal
16 to 30 μmol/L	Abnormal
31 to 100 μmol/L	Abnormal
Above 100 μmol/L	Abnormal

μmol/L = micromoles per liter

While no studies have adequately determined whether lowering homocysteine levels will help to reduce strokes, heart attacks, and other cardiovascular events, it is a good idea to lower your homocysteine level because of the known risk of heart disease with high levels of this amino acid.

You can do that by eating more fruits and vegetables (especially leafy green vegetables) and breakfast cereals, lentils, chickpeas, asparagus, and most beans. Be sure to take a multivitamin that includes about 1 mg of folate and vitamin B6 and vitamin B12 supplements. If taking these additional supplementary vitamins does not lower your homocysteine level, your doctor may have you try higher vitamin doses.

Check for Infections

You should always be on the lookout for chronic infections such as herpes, gum disease, lyme disease, and other diseases that cause inflammation. Treat as necessary with antibiotics, antiviral drugs, or other drugs recommended by your doctor, in order to reduce the amount of immunoglobulins and therefore decrease the viscosity of the blood. Aspirin and other anti-inflammatory drugs also may help. It may be that even chronic allergies play a role in increasing viscosity; only further studies will tell.

Note: Tylenol (acetaminophen) is not an anti-inflammatory and does not improve blood flow. It isn't a substitute for aspirin.

Other Cardiovascular Tests

In addition to general physicals, blood pressure measures, and blood tests, I think everyone should have several heart-specific tests. Ideally, you should have these during adolescence, but you should certainly get checked out if you're over forty or ready to begin any form of physical exercise. These tests include:

- treadmill test (or "stress test")
- electrocardiogram (ECG)
- echocardiogram

These tests must be ordered by your doctor. At present, a cardiologist is the only type of doctor that I know of who offers the stress test and the echocardiogram on a regular basis.

Stress Test

Cardiologists use a number of stress tests to measure how your heart and blood vessels respond to exercise. The most common is known as a treadmill exercise stress test (also called an exercise tolerance test or a stress electrocardiogram), a reliable, safe test which costs about $200. Before you start any exercise program, you should have a treadmill exercise stress test, even if your blood pressure is normal. Some people, including athletes (especially African Americans), experience dangerous blood pressure spikes during exercise. A stress test will help identify electrical abnormalities and blood pressure problems.

Before the Test You shouldn't eat, drink, smoke, or have any caffeine for four hours before the test. (Remember, coffee, tea, chocolate, cola drinks, and some over-the-counter pain relievers contain caffeine.) If you have diabetes, ask your doctor what you may eat. You should also tell the cardiologist about any medications you currently take.

The entire test takes about forty-five minutes. At least three electrodes on your chest and back will be wired to an electrocardiograph to record your heart's electrical activity. Before the test, the doctor will take a resting electrocardiogram (ECG), a blood pressure reading, and pulse levels. The ECG electrodes are kept in place as you exercise. Once you're walking on the treadmill, the doctor will increase the speed and incline every two to three minutes. If you're at high risk for coronary artery disease or in poor physical condition, the grade and speed may be increased in smaller increments. While you exercise, your doctor or a technician will look for changes in ECG patterns and blood pressure levels that may indicate that your heart isn't getting enough oxygen, as well as chest pain and unusual shortness of breath. It's normal to feel tired, to sweat, and to have some shortness of breath during testing. Your doctor will stop the test early if it is unsafe for you to continue.

You should tell the doctor if you feel any of the following symptoms during the test:

- chest, arm, or jaw discomfort
- severe shortness of breath
- fatigue
- dizziness
- leg cramps or soreness

Immediately after the test, you will be helped to a chair, where your heart rate and blood pressure are monitored for ten to fifteen minutes. You should wait at least one hour before you shower. Use warm water when showering because hot water may cause you to feel dizzy. You shouldn't start any exercise program until your doctor has reviewed the test results with you.

Side Effects This test places considerable stress on your heart. It may be hazardous if you have a heart aneurysm, uncontrolled disturbances in your heartbeat, inflammation of the sac surrounding your heart, inflammation of the heart muscle, severe anemia, uncontrolled high blood pressure, unstable angina, or congestive heart failure. Stop the test immediately if you experience any chest pain, extreme fatigue, or other complications.

Who Shouldn't Take a Stress Test   You shouldn't take an exercise stress test if you have any of the following conditions:

- severe congestive heart failure
- life-threatening abnormal heart rhythms
- heart infection
- severe valve disease
- severe high blood pressure

Electrocardiogram (ECG)

An electrocardiogram is a graphic recording of your heart's electrical activity. Electrical impulses move throughout the heart and play an important role in causing the heart to beat. An ECG can give your doctor lots of information about how healthy your heart is, including its rhythm, the chambers of your heart, the functioning of your heart muscle, and whether you had a heart attack in the past.

An ECG may be performed as part of a complete history and physical examination to provide a baseline picture of your heart's activity. Future ECGs can then highlight any changes or subsequent heart attack. The test is safe and painless; there are no known risks.

A health care practitioner will place electrodes on your body and attach the leads to the ECG machine. As you lie still, the technician will press a button to record your heart's electrical activity.

Echocardiogram

An echocardiogram is a painless diagnostic test that uses high-frequency sound waves (ultrasound) to obtain pictures of your heart. It can reveal any coronary artery disease and determine safe levels of exercise, especially if you have angina or other symptoms of coronary disease or heart failure. I think it's a good idea for every person to get a baseline echocardiogram in adolescence. This safe and painless test may help you avoid more risky, invasive diagnostic procedures later.

During the test, a trained technician uses a small, handheld device to produce the sound waves and receive the echoes as they "bounce" off the heart and reflect as images on a TV screen. The process doesn't involve exposure to radiation.

Echocardiography is considered one of the most powerful diagnostic tools in cardiology, since it can provide details about the anatomy of your heart and how it's working. The test can reveal the workings of your heart valves, how well your heart muscle moves, and how your blood flows. It can measure the dimensions of the four chambers of the heart and provide information about your arteries, as well as locate blood clots within the heart chambers.

If you're scheduling an exercise stress test for the same day as the echocardiogram, make sure you have the exercise test either after the echocardiogram or at least two to three hours before. That way, you can be sure the echocardiogram is performed under "at-rest" conditions.

The Body Shop of the Future

Twenty years ago, would you have thought that one day you could drive up to a local convenience store on a Sunday afternoon, walk over to a machine, swipe a card, and get a handful of cash?

Cash from a machine, on a Sunday? Of course not. Yet, today, just about everybody carries a bank card around to do just that. I predict that within ten years, you'll be stopping by your local pharmacist for a "tune-up in the body shop"—a quick evaluation of your cardiovascular system to monitor its efficiency. When you stop by to pick up a prescription, you'll be able to check your blood pressure, blood viscosity, heart contractility, and thirty to forty other measurements of blood characteristics. You'll sit down in a comfy lounge chair and lie back and watch TV or read a magazine as an assistant attaches a gadget to your arm that automatically finds your vein through ultrasound. After numbing the skin, the device will place a tiny needle in your vein automatically: you won't see or feel the needle, and you won't see the blood.

Within about fifteen minutes, your pharmacist will have your blood reading, including viscosity and other biophysical properties, C-reactive protein, electrolytes, enzymes, hematocrit (concentration of red blood cells), liver enzymes, homocysteine, and blood fat levels, as well as results of a battery of other chemical tests. All these studies will not only help to determine how efficient your heart is working but will scan for other diseases as well.

In the future, you may also wear an implantable blood pressure monitoring device, a watchlike device on your wrist that measures your blood pressure twenty times a second, together with a measurement of the force of your heart's contraction. When you visit the body shop of the future, the pharmacist can download the information from the past month from the blood pressure watch; if your heart isn't working efficiently, the doctor will have all the information to immediately prescribe individualized treatment.

In the body shop of the future, your doctor may also treat you with a new implantable device that can be programmed to help you lose a certain number of calories per day by urinating blood fats. The S.L.I.M. device, now under development, would be implanted in the chest much like a pacemaker and used as a means of weight control for very obese people or patients with severe hereditary blood fat abnormalities.

If your viscosity is high, or if your blood is too sticky, your pharmacist can give a quick call to your doctor for up-to-the-minute prescription alterations. You could have a half pint of blood drawn right there to reduce the viscosity. Blood pressure too high? You could have medication available right away to bring it down. Blood too sticky? Your physician will prescribe the latest lubricant.

Of course, this is all in the future. It may sound unbelievable, but to a citizen of the nineteenth century, how believable were jet planes? In 1915, who could have imagined a machine that cooks potatoes in a few minutes . . . that a thin, four-inch disk could contain an entire album of songs . . . or that one day, people all over the world would be able to communicate effortlessly and instantaneously, with words, pictures, sounds, and movement, over a telephone line?

Until the day comes when you can have a tune-up in the body shop, you can follow my simple, inexpensive seven-step plan to help you take control of your health and prevent (or reverse) blocked, hardened arteries.

Part 2

The Seven-Step Plan to Artery Health

6

For now, the easiest way to thin your blood and make it healthier is to donate blood every eight weeks, as recommended by the American Red Cross. Not only will donating your blood help make your blood thinner, but also your blood pressure will probably drop as the squeezing force of the left ventricle falls, easing the wear and tear on your arteries.

We've already seen stunning evidence from Finland in which men who gave blood were *four times* less likely to have heart attacks. Other studies have found similar results, claiming from a two- to tenfold reduction in heart attacks among men who gave blood. These researchers believe that blood donation helped lower the risk of heart attacks because it reduced iron levels in the body, which they think is somehow related to atherosclerosis. But, as discussed in the first chapters, iron can't be the cause of atherosclerosis, since iron itself doesn't explain why arteries become blocked only at certain sites, nor does it explain the connection with other risk factors such as diabetes or smoking.

It's far more likely that donating blood simply lowers blood thickness, for all the reasons already cited. Just remember: it's simple, it's safe, it costs nothing, and not only will you be helping yourself, but you could be saving another's life as well.

Why It Works

The thickness of your blood is determined mostly by the concentration and flexibility of the red blood cells. When you donate blood, you are temporarily lowering the concentration of the red blood cells. Donating blood speeds up the spleen's removal of red blood cells and removes blood cells when they are still flexible and less likely to cause injury to blood vessels. This causes the body to churn out *new* red blood cells that are young, healthy, and extremely flexible. You are making your blood thinner, less viscous, and it will flow more easily. You really get a "three-for-one": thinning your blood (1) decreases the work of the heart, (2) increases the ease with which the blood flows and reaches all of your other organs (the brain as well), and (3) reduces the risk of developing atherosclerosis. This is especially important for men, who have a higher concentration of red blood cells to start with, which raises their natural blood viscosity by about 25 percent. This means that a man's heart is already working 25 percent harder, so his arteries take 25 percent more of a beating with each pulse.

Tips from the Racetrack

Racehorse breeders have been using this technique (they call it "blood doping" around the track) since about 1910. Breeders discovered that if they removed blood from a racehorse and then let the horse recover for a few days, the horse would run much faster than it could before. Those in the racing world thought this was because removing blood somehow made the blood thicker. It turns out that the racehorse owners were pretty smart—blood doping worked, but not because it thickened blood. After blood doping, the animal had thinner, less viscous blood, and its heart didn't have to work so hard.

The same thing happens when we donate blood. Having your red blood cells removed on a regular basis is a key factor in tuning up your blood, just as changing the oil in your car every 5,000 miles will keep your engine working in top condition for a much longer period of time.

Who Should Give Blood?

Almost anyone who isn't menstruating or pregnant will probably benefit from giving blood. Certainly, if you have very thick blood, high blood pressure, diabetes, heart disease, or a heart that's squeezing with too much force, you'll be much better off if you donate regularly. In particular, all men, obese people, stroke patients, and postmenopausal women are prime candidates for donating to thin the blood. In addition, patients with kidney disease or polycythemia vera (a rare disease of too many red blood cells) will also benefit from donating blood on a regular basis. Now that we can measure blood viscosity, we can show that keeping viscosity below a certain level can stop atherosclerosis.

How Often?

If you're healthy and you weigh at least 110 pounds, you can donate a pint of blood every eight weeks, according to American Red Cross guidelines. (Some states may further limit the number or frequency of donations in a twelve-month period.)

Someday, we expect that when we measure and monitor each person's blood viscosity and other blood flow characteristics, we'll be able to develop an individually tailored schedule for blood donations that will keep the heart working at its greatest efficiency with the least amount of effort and turbulence. Until then, it's safe to go by the Red Cross guidelines.

Donate Blood, Lower Fat Levels

I think we'll also find that when we lower the blood's thickness by donating blood more often than every eight weeks, we can also lower blood fats—at least, the levels won't rise. It's not too much of a stretch to imagine that treatments like blood donation may also be an effective means of lowering blood fats without using drugs.

Can Everyone Donate Blood?

Red Cross guidelines stipulate that to give blood, you must be healthy, at least seventeen years old, and weigh at least 110 pounds. If you're over age sixty-five and in good health, you can usually donate with the approval of the blood bank physician.

If you have a cold or the flu, or if you're pregnant or you've recently had a baby, surgery, or serious illness, you may be temporarily deferred. You can still give blood if you take medication, depending on the type and the condition for which it was prescribed. Consult your doctor or the blood center medical staff if you have questions about your eligibility to donate.

If you've recently traveled to Africa, Central America, or South America in places with high concentrations of certain diseases (such as malaria), you may be unable to donate blood for about a year. If you've been vaccinated for measles, mumps, and rubella, you may not be able to donate for about a month.

If you recently got a tattoo, you must wait a year before donating blood. (It doesn't matter how many tattoos you have, just when you got the last one.) You can still give blood if you've had your body pierced, if it was done by a licensed professional. Nonprofessional body piercing prevents you from giving blood for about one year.

Storing Your Own Blood

If you know you'll be having surgery soon, you can donate blood for your own use; doctors call this "autologous" blood donation. There are three types of autologous procedures available:

- preoperative donation: donating your own blood prior to the surgery
- intraoperative donation: saving blood lost during surgery for return to you
- postoperative cell salvage: saving your blood lost immediately after surgery for return to you

Donate for Research

If you can't donate your blood to give to others and you aren't planning on having any surgeries, you may be able to donate your blood to the American Red Cross research blood donor program. Blood is needed for medical research by scientists at the American Red Cross Holland Laboratory in Rockville, Maryland. Because blood for research can't be taken from the national transfusion blood supply, special donors are recruited for the purpose. Research donors should be healthy individuals who have been deferred from donating blood for any of a variety of reasons. The scientists are looking for donors who have:

FOR MORE INFORMATION . . .

For more information about donating blood for research, contact:

Research Blood Program Coordinator
Holland Laboratory
15601 Crabbs Branch Way
Rockville, MD 20855
(301) 738-0471

- taken antimalarial medications
- tested positive for hepatitis
- had cancer and been in remission for more than two years

Blood from these donors is used for a variety of research studies, such as looking for ways to remove viruses from the blood, studying blood cell functions, and developing better methods to process, store, and ship blood components.

Who Can't Donate to Give to Others?

There are some people in certain risk groups who are not allowed to donate blood to give to others; however, if you fall into one of these risk groups, you can still donate blood to be stored and used for your own benefit.

While specific rules may vary from one state to another, in general, you are prohibited from donating your blood to give to others if you:

- have used illegal intravenous drugs, even once
- are a man who has had sex with another man since 1977, even once

- have hemophilia
- have ever had a positive antibody test for HIV (AIDS virus)
- are a man or woman who has had sex for money or drugs anytime since 1977
- have had hepatitis anytime after your eleventh birthday
- have ever had cancer (except localized skin cancer)
- have multiple sclerosis
- have had myocardial infarction or coronary artery bypass surgery
- have had a stroke
- have had babesiosis or Chagas' disease
- have taken Tegison for psoriasis
- have Creutzfeldt-Jakob disease (CJD) or a member of your immediate family has CJD
- have had live animal tissue or cell transplants

Is It Safe?

Each needle used in the procedure is sterile and is disposed of after a single use. It's not possible to contract HIV (the virus that causes AIDS) or any other disease by donating blood.

Where to Donate

There are many places where you can donate blood. Bloodmobiles travel to high schools, colleges, churches, and other community organizations. You also can donate at community blood centers and hospital-based donor centers. Many people donate at blood drives at the workplace. With luck, ways to donate and the number of centers will expand in the future. To find out where you can donate, call (800) 448-3543 or contact your local Red Cross.

Before You Donate

Blood donation experts offer these tips to follow the day before you donate blood:

- Don't take aspirin (or products containing aspirin) for at least seventy-two hours before your scheduled appointment.
- Get a good night's sleep.
- Eat at your regular mealtimes.
- Drink plenty of fluids several hours before you donate.
- Eat breakfast.
- Relax.

What to Expect

Because of the risk of infectious diseases in donated blood, donors are carefully recruited and screened for health risk factors. The Red Cross makes every effort to recruit a healthy population of volunteer blood donors; 2 percent of the blood it collects is discarded because of uncertain test results.

The donation process has six stages, as follows.

1. Schedule an Appointment.

The average blood donation process takes about one hour from start to finish; the actual donation takes six to ten minutes.

2. Register to Donate.

Arrive at your appointed time with picture identification and social security information.

3. Complete Medical Screening.

A medical professional will take your vital signs and ask you questions about your general medical health and lifestyle in a private setting. The Food and Drug Administration (FDA) has established stringent guidelines that donors must meet. It's during this process that you may be temporarily or permanently deferred. All information remains confidential.

You'll first be given an introductory pamphlet about donating blood, the infections that can be transmitted by donor blood (especially HIV), and the risk behaviors associated with those infections. People who think they may be at risk are asked not to donate. After you read the pamphlet, a trained, qualified professional will conduct the confidential interview with you, taking a health history and asking direct questions about high-risk behaviors, including intravenous drug use, sex with intravenous drug users, and male-to-male sexual contact. If you answer yes to any of these questions, you will be deferred indefinitely, in accordance with FDA guidelines.

If you answer no to all the questions, you will be asked to sign a statement confirming that you have read and understood the information and the questions asked and that you aren't engaged in any of the high-risk behaviors for HIV.

You also receive a "confidential unit exclusion" (CUE) form. High-risk donors who may not wish to reveal risk behaviors privately to the nurse may confidentially exclude their donated blood by peeling a bar code sticker off the CUE form and placing it on the donation record. A computer reads the code as "do not transfuse," instructing the Red Cross staff to discard that unit of blood.

You will be given a telephone number to call within twenty-four hours and a special identification code to use if for any reason, after leaving the donation site, you decide that your blood should not be used.

In addition to maintaining local records that identify all unsuitable donors, the Red Cross has been maintaining a national computerized database of more than 250,000 donors who are deferred from donating blood due to a history of risk-associated behavior, signs or symptoms that could be associated with various transmissible diseases, or a positive result for any of the viruses tested. Every donation received by the Red Cross is cross-checked against these Red Cross deferred donor databases to determine if the blood should be destroyed based on past test results.

Your blood will be tested for evidence of transmissible diseases. Every unit of blood is tested for evidence of exposure to viruses that may cause diseases, including HIV, two strains of hepatitis, HTLV (human T-cell leukemia/lymphoma virus), and syphilis. If there's no problem, it can be used either as whole blood for one patient or, after separation into components, to help several patients. If testing indicates that a unit of blood may pose a threat, it is destroyed. The donor is disqualified and entered in the deferred donor database. Counseling is available for donors who are deferred from donating blood, whether temporarily or permanently, due to positive results on any of the tests.

4. Your Blood Donation.

A skilled, specially trained medical technician will clean your arm and use a sterilized needle to draw blood. The procedure takes six to ten minutes. All materials used for your donation are new, sterile, disposable, and used only once; there is no chance of contracting AIDS or any other communicable disease from donating blood. There may be a little sting when the needle is inserted, but there should be no pain during the procedure.

You will give a little less than one pint of whole blood. (The average adult has between eight and twelve pints of blood and can easily spare one.)

5. You're Done!

After you give blood, you'll be asked to stay at least ten minutes. During this time, you will be served refreshments, including juice and cookies, in order to raise your blood sugar and replenish your fluids.

6. Donate Again!

You may give the gift of life as often as every eight weeks.

After You Donate

Most people feel great after the donation. Donors who know what to expect and have eaten regular meals before donating are usually fine. After spending about an hour at the donation site, you can resume full activity as long as you feel good. Just avoid lifting, pushing, or picking up heavy objects for at least four or five hours after giving blood. Don't smoke for thirty minutes after donating. Drink extra fluids for the next forty-eight hours—but no alcoholic beverages! Eat a hearty meal. If you feel faint or dizzy, either sit down with your head between your knees or lie down with your head lower than the rest of your body. You may remove the Band-Aid after twenty-four hours. Your body replaces blood volume, or plasma, within twenty-four hours, but it takes four to eight weeks for red blood cells to be replaced.

7

Step Two:
An Aspirin a Day

Most of us have used aspirin to ease a pounding headache, but you can get much more benefit from aspirin than pain relief. A *daily low dose* of aspirin is an important part of a heart-healthy life. While you may already have heard that taking a tablet a day is "good for the heart," you may not understand *why*.

Aspirin is critical as a way to prevent coronary artery disease. As discussed in earlier chapters, in order to function properly, the heart must receive a constant, reliable flow of oxygen-rich blood. When this flow is restricted by narrowed arteries, it can lead to a heart attack (the death of a portion of heart muscle). Many people think of aspirin as a blood thinner, but this isn't quite accurate.

In early studies, scientists have found that aspirin makes a dramatic difference in the blood's clotting potential. Basically, aspirin is a drug that stops platelets from sticking to injured surfaces, keeping them from clumping together as they normally do to form blood clots at sites of injury. Once aspirin affects a platelet in this way, it can never become sticky again.

In the future, we will be able to quantify dosages for each individual patient, as well as find other drugs that may be more effective than aspirin. In the meantime, it is a very inexpensive way to help prevent major artery blockages.

What does this mean for your arteries? It means that when you take aspirin, you're stopping the formation of calluses (plaques) at the sites where the turbulent blood is injuring the walls of the arteries. Taking an aspirin is like coating a ski with wax; it keeps the ski running smoothly.

In one Harvard University study, one aspirin every other day cut the heart attack risk in half. When taken during (or immediately after) a heart attack, aspirin appears to significantly reduce the risk of death during the first five weeks after the attack. Aspirin will also reduce the chance of your blood vessels blocking up again after bypass graft surgery.

The wonderful thing about aspirin is that it can be so effective at such a low price: one generic aspirin tablet a day costs just pennies. After you brush your teeth every morning, you should routinely take your aspirin.

Inflammation and Aspirin

More recent research suggests a link between viruses (especially CMV, a member of the herpes family) and atherosclerosis, an idea that supports the role of inflammation in the plaque-forming process. When there is inflammation in the body (especially long-term inflammation), the blood gets thicker and more viscous. This is why people with inflammatory conditions, including arthritis, allergies, asthma, lupus, and frequent viral or bacterial infections, would benefit from taking a daily aspirin tablet. Aspirin reduces inflammatory responses of the

IF YOU THINK YOU'RE HAVING A HEART ATTACK . . .

If you suspect that you are having a heart attack, seek emergency medical care immediately, and then take an aspirin. You'll likely do no harm by taking the aspirin, and you'll have a great chance of helping yourself.

body to infection and injury. Theoretically at least, aspirin should reduce the quantity of antibodies and immunoglobulins in the blood and therefore reduce blood thickness.

Who Can Benefit

Nearly all people can benefit from taking a once-a-day low-dose aspirin. In general, taking an aspirin once a day is cheap; it's easy; and for the most part, it can't hurt. In fact, if you are in the process of having a heart attack, an aspirin may help quell it. If your current medical condition or medical history includes any of the following, you should take an aspirin daily:

- heart attack
- angina (chest pain from poor blood supply to the heart) or claudication (leg pain from poor blood supply to the legs)
- bypass graft surgery or balloon angioplasty for diseased arteries of the heart or legs
- stroke
- temporary "ministroke" (TIA: transient ischemic attack)
- disturbed heart rhythm known as atrial fibrillation

Those who may benefit most from the preventive effects of aspirin are men over forty and menopausal women who:

- can't stop smoking
- have high blood fats or high blood pressure
- have a family history of heart attack, stroke, or other blood vessel disease
- are obese
- have diabetes

Who Should Not Take Aspirin

While the U.S. Food and Drug Administration recognizes that aspirin regimen helps reduce the risk of stroke or heart attacks for certain people (such as those who have already had a heart attack), it can in rare cases cause other health problems. These include prolonged bleeding, ulcers, and allergic reaction. (People with sensitive stomachs may want to take buffered aspirin.)

Pregnant women should not take low-dose aspirin without consulting a doctor. Also, you should not take aspirin if you:

- have had problems with aspirin
- are allergic to aspirin or other salicylates
- are an alcoholic
- have a stomach or duodenal ulcer (take coated aspirin instead)
- have stomach bleeding
- have any bleeding disorder or a general tendency to bleed
- have uncontrolled high blood pressure
- have severe liver or kidney disease

The Downside

There is a downside to altering the stickiness of platelets: if you do have a stroke, or an artery breaks in your brain, you'll be more likely to die if you've been taking daily doses of aspirin. *But you have a far greater chance of having fatal problems with atherosclerosis than of dying from a ruptured artery in the brain.* In fact, aspirin is so important to your heart's health that I recommend that teenagers start taking an aspirin a day for life.

Although many experts suspect that anti-inflammatory drugs such as ibuprofen (Motrin or Advil), naproxen sodium, and ketoprofen will work just as well as aspirin in reducing the stickiness of platelets, research has not yet proved this. These drugs, like aspirin, treat pain and fever effectively, but up to this point, only aspirin has demonstrated a beneficial effect for heart attack and stroke, and it does reduce inflammation.

You *cannot* simply substitute Tylenol (acetaminophen) for aspirin; it does not work in the same way as does aspirin, nor has it been shown to have any of the heart benefits, and it does not reduce inflammation. Many people think that Tylenol and aspirin are the same; they aren't. A note of warning: Tylenol (acetaminophen) taken every day for several years can destroy your kidneys.

Side Effects

Aspirin is generally very safe, but like all other drugs, it can have side effects, and in a small minority of people, it may be dangerous. The following side effects and risks are very low if you're taking the small, 80 mg dose. Again, in the future, this dosage should be individualized for each person. If you have blood vessel or heart disease, the potential benefits usually far outweigh the risk of having a stroke.

Rare side effects include:

- heartburn (Take enteric-coated aspirin to avoid this. It is designed to be absorbed in the intestine so it doesn't burn the stomach.)
- stomach pain (Take coated aspirin to avoid this.)
- minor bleeding from the stomach
- worsening of duodenal or stomach ulcers (In such cases, coated aspirin may help.)
- very slight risk of a stroke from bleeding in the brain

People who consume three or more alcoholic drinks every day should realize that there are bleeding risks involved with chronic, heavy alcohol use while taking aspirin.

How Much to Take

Further studies will probably show that some people will need more than others. But as far as we know now, you don't need to take megadoses of aspirin in order to get health benefits. In fact, you should be careful not to take large amounts of aspirin. (In this case, more is *not* better.)

For prevention of artery damage, the present recommended daily dose is 75 to 150 mg; typically, most people aim for about 80 mg a day. (A standard aspirin tablet is 300 to 325 mg.) Higher doses give no more benefits that we can measure at the present time, but they do have more side effects.

The smaller 80 mg dose is an amount that is found in one tablet of "children's" aspirin. Today, you can find this dose sold in special tablets marketed for those taking the medication for heart purposes; for example, Bayer sells a product called Aspirin Regimen at 81 mg doses, with calcium. (You won't see specific recommendations on the bottle about taking aspirin for the heart, however; the FDA doesn't yet allow aspirin manufacturers to make claims about heart disease prevention on their labels.)

When doctors or ambulance staff suspect that someone is having a heart attack, they will advise a higher dose of half to one 325 mg tablet taken straight away (preferably the type that can be dissolved in water).

Numerous studies both in the United States and abroad have established the safety and efficacy of aspirin in preventing heart attacks and strokes.

Is Aspirin Enough?

Aspirin alone will not prevent cardiovascular disease. The other factors that cause atherosclerosis—high blood pressure, high blood viscosity, and the force of the heart's contraction—can't be controlled or reversed by taking aspirin. Aspirin only stops the platelets from starting the process of callus formation. The only way to help prevent coronary artery disease is to develop a heart that pumps efficiently. Taking aspirin is only one part of the heart-healthy plan. You'll need to follow the rest of the seven-step plan to keep your arteries healthy. Make that commitment.

Ask Your Doctor

Always check with your doctor before taking any medication. And, remember that no drug, not even aspirin, can single-handedly prevent heart disease. Your personal commitment to getting your heart to pump efficiently is your best defense against heart disease.

8

Step Three:
Try to Stop Smoking

Of all the risks that are linked with hardening of the arteries, smoking is perhaps the most critical because it increases all three factors that determine the work of the heart: blood thickness, blood pressure, and the squeezing force of the heart's left ventricle. Fortunately, smoking is one risk factor that you can eliminate right away—and the benefit lasts forever.

Smoking is extremely addictive (some say more than heroin). Most people know that smoking is bad for the lungs, but not very many people understand how it can affect the arteries. Doctors have known for a long time that smoking is one of the main contributors to hardening of the arteries. The stimulating effects of nicotine in cigarettes causes major constriction of the small arteries, boosting blood pressure and increasing the squeezing force of the heart. This puts you at a higher risk for heart attack and stroke. Smoking also decreases the oxygen carried in the blood.

Without a doubt, smoking increases the viscosity of the blood by raising the concentration of red blood cells, and the tars in cigarette smoke also make the blood stickier. When most people think of tars, they think of lung damage, but tar doesn't just stay in the lungs. Some goes into the blood and mixes with plasma, increasing the viscosity and stickiness of the blood. This makes the blood thicker by increasing the concentration of red blood cells. (The carbon monoxide from smoke attaches itself to a red blood cell, preventing that cell from carrying oxygen.) Therefore, the body has to make more red blood cells to make up for the ones that no longer work. And since the concentration of red blood cells (hematocrit) is crucial in determining how thick your blood is, the more you smoke, the thicker your blood will become.

Smoking and Other Risk Factors

What's worse, smoking interacts with other risk factors to further increase your chances for developing artery disease. Cigarette smoking is responsible for between 17 percent and 30 percent of all deaths from cardiovascular illness.

Any amount of smoking is dangerous. Even if you smoke only one to four cigarettes a day, you're significantly increasing your risk of someday developing atherosclerosis. Moreover, the effects of cigarette smoking are dose related. Women who smoke more than twenty-five cigarettes per day are five times more likely to eventually suffer from atherosclerosis than nonsmokers.

Smoking and High Blood Pressure

If you already have high blood pressure, smoking will dramatically increase your chances of getting cardiovascular disease. The nicotine in cigarettes temporarily increases your heart rate and blood pressure and raises the heart's oxygen requirements. At the same time, the carbon monoxide in smoke lowers the amount of oxygen in the circulating blood, reducing the oxygen going to various parts of the body (including the heart), just when it's most needed.

Secondhand Smoke

Unfortunately, smoking isn't hurting just the person puffing on the cigarette; it's also endangering friends and family members. In fact, the American Heart Association estimates that every year, up to 40,000 people die from heart and blood vessel disease caused by passive smoking.

Secondhand smoke is that gray cloud you see wafting away from a burning cigarette between puffs that gets inhaled not just by the smoker but also by everyone else in the smoker's vicinity. This secondhand smoke contains many of the same harmful components inhaled by the smoker—and it actually contains more of some compounds (such as carbon monoxide) that interfere with the delivery of oxygen to the heart.

How much secondhand smoke you're exposed to is important in determining how much of a health risk you face. For example, if someone you live with smokes, there's a significant association between the

CIGAR SMOKING

Experts don't agree on whether smoking cigars increases your risk for coronary artery disease; some believe it may be less likely to impair your arteries because cigar smokers are less likely to inhale. Until proved otherwise, cigars have the same risk of causing artery disease as cigarettes, for all the same reasons.

number of cigarettes he or she smokes each day and your own risk of heart attack: if your cohabitant smokes more than twenty cigarettes a day, *you* have four times the risk of a heart attack.

But it's not just the passive smoke you inhale in the home that could be hurting you; passive smoking at work is just about as dangerous as the exposure to such smoke at home. And just as in active smoking, passive smoking affects other coronary risk factors such as hypertension, family history of heart attack, and diabetes.

Will Quitting Help?

If you quit smoking and avoid exposure to secondhand smoke, you'll immediately reduce your risk of heart attack, and within one year of quitting, your risk of developing coronary artery disease will be cut in half. Three or four years after quitting, your risk of artery disease is about the same as that of people who have never smoked. *Research has shown that quitting smoking will lower your risk of artery disease no matter how old you are.*

Within twelve hours of smoking your last cigarette, the levels of carbon monoxide and nicotine in your system begin to fall rapidly, according to the National Cancer Society. Your heart and lungs will begin to heal. But don't be surprised if you don't immediately feel better; in fact, you may feel worse at first. You should expect to undergo temporary withdrawal symptoms. *They won't last.*

When you quit, you may experience:

- slowed metabolism
- weight gain
- irregularity
- dry, sore gums or tongue
- edgy, angry, grumpy feelings
- hunger
- fatigue

- sleeping problems
- coughing

Although your body will get rid of nicotine in two to three days, you may continue to experience withdrawal symptoms for one to two weeks. Within a few days, your sense of taste and smell may improve. You'll breathe more easily.

Tips from the Experts

There is no magical approach to quitting that works for everybody, according to government experts at the National Institute of Drug Abuse (NIDA) and the U.S. Food and Drug Administration (FDA). There are plenty of things you can do right away to help yourself stop smoking and deal with the urges. In addition, you may find that a combination of nicotine-replacement therapy (gum, patches, or sprays), medication, and behavioral support will be your best bet for success, according to NIDA experts.

The following tips are adapted from information provided by the National Cancer Institute, the National Heart, Lung, and Blood Institute, and NIDA.

1. Set a "quit date" now, and write it down somewhere so that you can see the date approaching. Try quitting during a vacation—it may be easier.
2. Get support from others when you decide to quit: tell someone; join a support group.
3. Throw away your cigarettes and matches. Hide your lighters and ashtrays.
4. Have your teeth cleaned by the dentist.
5. Buy flowers. Enjoy the scent.
6. If you decide to taper off instead of quitting cold turkey, switch to a brand you find distasteful.

7. Alter your routine, to avoid the urge to smoke.
8. Drink plenty of water to manage withdrawal more effectively, or drink milk (some find it unpleasant with smoking).
9. Substitute sugarless gum, carrot sticks, or low-calorie candies to control the urge to smoke.
10. Get up from the table after eating, and brush your teeth immediately.
11. Keep your hands busy with keys, coins, or worry beads.
12. Make your home and car smoke-free.
13. Get plenty of rest.
14. Use positive thinking.
15. Learn relaxation techniques.
16. Ask your doctor about ways to quit smoking.

Nicotine Replacement

Nicotine is a psychoactive drug that induces euphoria, according to NIDA; when you stop smoking, the euphoria goes away. Nicotine-replacement therapy will ease some of the withdrawal symptoms associated with this loss of euphoria and thus reduce your craving for cigarettes. However, don't think that nicotine replacement won't increase your risk for coronary artery disease. While it's much better than smoking, nicotine is still a potent heart stimulant and artery constrictor.

For many people, this approach is an answer to handling the cravings and withdrawal from nicotine. If you're quitting, it's one avenue to consider. However, pregnant or breast-feeding women should not use nicotine in any form. You also should not use these products if you have cardiovascular disease or asthma. There are other considerations that you should discuss with your doctor, including any potential risks.

At the moment, there are three types of replacement therapy: nicotine gum, nicotine patches (prescription and nonprescription), and nicotine nasal spray.

Nicotine Gum

When you chew nicotine gum, you release nicotine into your body. If you were a pack-a-day smoker (or more), chewing the gum will ease the discomfort of withdrawal but won't get rid of the symptoms completely. You'll also get some of the euphoric effect of nicotine but less than with cigarettes.

To get the best effects, you must chew the gum slowly; when you get a peppery sensation, you should then park the gum between your cheek and gums. At first, this may cause hiccups, upset stomach, or aching jaw. If you chew correctly, however, most of the side effects will go away. It usually takes three to six months to wean yourself from the nicotine gum.

Nicotine Patches

Nicotine patches deliver nicotine to the blood in your veins through your skin. As with the gum, withdrawal symptoms are less intense but won't be completely eliminated. Each day, you should remove the old patch and place a new one somewhere on your body between your neck and your waist. Patches come in different doses and also in full-dose or tapering-dose programs. Ask your doctor which is best for you. The full-dose program usually lasts six weeks.

Some people get a mild rash under the patch, which is easily treated. It may help to move the patch to another part of your body. If you use the patches at night, you may experience vivid dreams or other sleep problems.

A nonprescription, over-the-counter version of the nicotine patch was approved in April 2000. Called Clear NicoDerm CQ, this clear patch works the same way as the original NicoDerm CQ, by relieving withdrawal symptoms and providing a temporary source of nicotine. The product is available in the same strengths as the original nicotine patch. While it is available over the counter, you should consult a doctor if you have asthma, heart disease, a recent history of heart attack, uncontrolled high blood pressure, or irregular heartbeat, since the product can increase your heart rate and blood pressure. You should also consult your doctor before using this product if you are taking any antidepressants.

Nicotine Nasal Spray

A nicotine nasal spray (Nicotrol NS), approved by the FDA in 1996, is considered to be as effective as nicotine gum or patches. Like these products, the nasal spray reduces craving and withdrawal symptoms, allowing smokers to cut back gradually. The spray allows nicotine to be inhaled through your nose and into your bloodstream, replacing the nicotine you would otherwise get from smoking. In this way, the withdrawal effects are less severe. As your body adjusts to the loss of cigarettes, the use of the spray is decreased gradually over several weeks and finally stopped.

The nasal spray has some advantages over the gum and the patch: because the nicotine is quickly absorbed across the nasal membranes,

WARNING

Smoking during nicotine-replacement therapy can be dangerous, as the level of nicotine in your body can rise to toxic levels. It's also likely that smoking during treatment will sabotage your efforts to quit permanently.

CUTTING BACK VERSUS QUITTING

Cutting back may help you as a way of practicing quitting, but it probably won't reduce your health risks because most smokers who cut back inhale more often and more deeply. This means that even though you seem to be smoking fewer cigarettes, you really haven't cut back at all. The same situation occurs when you switch to low-tar or low-nicotine cigarettes.

it has a quick, strong effect more like a cigarette. Unfortunately, the fact that it works so quickly means there's a bigger risk for addiction than with the slower-acting gum and patch. The manufacturer estimates that the addiction potential is about midway between that of smoking itself and using the gum or patch. Some reports suggest that hard-core smokers are eight times more likely to quit smoking using the spray than using patches.

Smoking-Cessation Medications

A prescription antidepressant called bupropion (trade names: Wellbutrin or Zyban) has been shown to be effective in helping people quit, according to the FDA. Effects of bupropion include dry mouth and insomnia; if you have a preexisting seizure disorder, anorexia nervosa, or bulimia, your chances for a seizure increase while on bupropion. Higher doses of bupropion seem to work better than lower doses and also may decrease the weight gain that often occurs when you try to stop smoking.

You should avoid amphetamines if you're trying to quit smoking; they may actually increase your smoking habit.

Relapses

Most relapses occur in the first week of quitting, according to the National Institute of Drug Abuse; most of the rest happen in the first three months. Usually, something specific sets off a return to the smoking habit. If you can anticipate potential triggers, you may be able to resist. According to NIDA, potential triggers include:

- work pressure
- eating
- drinking alcoholic or caffeinated beverages
- talking on the phone
- being around smokers
- playing cards or games
- deadline pressure
- getting into an argument
- feelings of sadness or frustration

If you have a relapse, don't despair. Smoking is one of the most difficult habits to break—some say more difficult than withdrawal from illegal drugs such as heroin or cocaine. Most ex-smokers tried to quit several times before they finally succeeded.

9

You've been poring over those reports all morning, watching the clock with one eye as you highlight and underline. You don't feel thirsty, so your body must be doing just fine on that orange juice and cup of coffee you grabbed at home two hours ago, right? Wrong.

Most people think that the sensation of thirst is your body's way of telling you it needs fluids, but that's not true. Once you realize you're thirsty, you're already dehydrated. You need to drink enough water so that you don't *get* thirsty in the first place—just as you should keep your car topped up with oil instead of waiting for the red oil-warning light to come on. You may not realize that you don't lose water just when you urinate; every minute, as you breathe, sweat, and move around, you're losing water into the atmosphere. That fluid must be replaced.

Water has no effect on your body until it's passed into the gastrointestinal tract and on into the blood. Along the way, the kidney is in constant control of the proportion of essential salts dissolved in blood. It's the balance between your body fluids and these dissolved salt particles that tells the brain just how dry you are. In turn, the brain sends the body other signals, such as decreased saliva flow, that tell you when you're thirsty. However, you may have all the right critical concentrations of salt dissolved in your blood to live and have very high or low viscosity. No organ in your body directly monitors or controls your blood viscosity.

When it comes to your heart, drinking plenty of water actually lowers blood pressure, softens and liquefies blood cells, and helps the cells move through your arteries more easily. With further research, I believe we'll find that fluids play a far more important role in blood viscosity than we ever realized. And yet, while water is critical to keeping the blood thin and flowing smoothly, the thirst sensation probably doesn't correlate with blood viscosity any more than with dehydration. You can go for hours without any fluid, to the point where your blood is getting as thick as molasses, and still you might not feel thirsty.

Water and Blood Pressure

Most people know that using a lot of salt will raise blood pressure. Yet, few people seem to realize that drinking enough water may help lower blood pressure. In fact, for many years, doctors prescribed diuretics (drugs that help you urinate) to lower blood pressure. Many studies have since shown that strokes were often the unfortunate consequence of this treatment. This isn't surprising when you consider that using diuretics will make blood much thicker, which could create or greatly accelerate the harmful process in the blood vessels. Most people are even less aware that water has the ability to lower the viscosity of your blood.

We don't know how blood viscosity varies throughout the day, but I suspect there is a big variation. It's a fact that you lose fluids when you breathe, perspire, and urinate. (That's why you may lose a little weight each night.) This could explain why heart attacks occur more often in the morning: you are dehydrated and therefore your blood is thicker. If you have dark, highly-concentrated urine when you wake up, it's a signal that your body is dehydrated. If this is happening to you, try to drink a few glasses of water at bedtime.

How Much Is Enough?

Your mother knew best: drinking six to ten glasses of water a day is good for you. I recommend even more: twelve glasses of water a day to keep your blood nice and thin. Unfortunately, I believe that most adults go through their entire lives in a basically dehydrated state.

Many people drink no water at all, and then compound the problem by turning to caffeinated or alcoholic beverages when they do drink. Caffeine and alcohol both have dehydrating effects that result in serious consequences for the body, not only in terms of kidney health and function, but also in terms of your blood pressure and blood viscosity. In fact, drinking enough water may be far more critical in determining your blood's viscosity than previously thought.

The good news is that drinking more water isn't going to hurt you. In fact, in terms of health benefits, few things can match water's extensive pedigree. Water benefits elimination and detoxification, and helps most of your body's systems work more efficiently. Drinking more water is one important way that you can begin—today—to lower your blood thickness with very little effort and no expense.

If you want to keep your arteries healthy and your blood thin, you need to take active responsibility for making sure your body gets enough fluids. You need to set a standard: I recommend twelve cups of fluid a day (about three quarts). Keep fluids at your bedside, at your desk, in your car.

If you have a weight problem, you'll need an extra cup of water for every twenty-five pounds of excess weight. In addition, you should increase the amount of water you drink if you exercise briskly or if the weather is hot and dry.

Special Concerns for Athletes

Coaches should be sure to have plenty of fluids on hand for their athletes, who are at special risk for dehydration because exercise, sweating, and even heavy breathing use up so much water. Athletes should never be thirsty; it's hard for an athlete to drink too much water when exercising. Choose a sports drink or plain water: just be sure to drink plenty.

Not Just Any Fluids

When I say "fluid," I really mean water. Can't stand plain water? Try a naturally carbonated water such as Perrier, which comes flavored with lemon and lime, too. Or reach for bottled spring water; you may find the taste is better than tap water.

If plain water really is unpalatable, seltzer water mixed with fruit juices is a pleasant, easy-to-prepare alternative. What's most important is to find a beverage that you enjoy drinking and that isn't high in calories or filled with stimulants or sugars—and no diet drinks! Diet drinks dehydrate. The artificial sugars can't be used by the body, so they are excreted by the kidney in the urine along with water. The result is that you lose more fluids than you drank in the first place.

In addition, avoid drinks with caffeine, such as colas, some root beers, and coffee. All of these stimulate the heart to contract harder.

Alcohol: Just Say No!

You are probably familiar with the research that found that moderate alcohol intake (one or two drinks a day) seems to lower the risk of heart attack and coronary heart disease. This is apparently true of all types of alcohol, including beer, white and red wine, and liquors. It is not clear why alcohol decreases the risk of heart attacks. I believe that alcohol's beneficial effects on the arteries have most to do with its ability to increase red blood cell flexibility when taken in very small amounts.

However, while one drink of alcohol may help lower atherosclerosis, alcohol in greater quantities raises blood fats and in high amounts also raises blood pressure. In some people, alcohol clearly has a dehydrating effect, and therefore, in these folks, it can considerably increase blood thickness. (This effect varies considerably from one person to the next, just as the ability to "hold your liquor" varies from person to person.)

Despite the benefits of one drink of alcohol on the arteries, I'm not recommending that anyone drink alcohol to help the arteries. In fact, I think it would be malpractice to recommend it, because it's human nature to assume that if one is good, then five is better.

Alcohol should never be used simply as a "medication" to prevent heart disease. There are just too many risks associated with drinking alcohol, from driving under the influence to an increased risk of liver disease or cancer. There's no getting around the fact that alcohol is a drug that has destroyed millions of lives, wrecked marriages and families, and killed innocent victims in drunk-driving accidents.

The decision to prescribe modest alcohol consumption as a preventive measure is not one that can be made without knowing your risk factors (including blood pressure, history, and triglyceride levels), your response to alcohol, and your addiction potential.

IO

You Are What You Eat

Whole forests have probably been cut down in the service of diet books, magazine articles, and newspaper pieces that explain the importance of a low-fat diet. There's no doubt that a low-fat diet (emphasizing fish, vegetables, and fruit) is your healthiest choice; your body works best with this type of fuel. Just as you wouldn't use diesel fuel in your car's gasoline engine, you shouldn't put animal fats into your system. There are nine calories in a gram of fat, but only four calories in a gram of carbohydrates or protein. The simplest way to improve artery health: don't eat fast food and fried food. Period.

Our society and its government have begun to take legal action against the huge tobacco companies that make astronomical profits by enticing people to smoke. What is even more perplexing is how huge corporations are making billions of dollars touting, pushing, glamorizing, and yes, rewarding our children with gifts of toys to eat foods that will accelerate the diseases that will kill more than 50 percent of them. These same corporate giants could instead spend their marketing and development millions in creating healthier foods and teaching our children to enjoy eating healthy meals.

It's just common sense: If you pour fat into your blood, it will get thicker. This makes it harder for your heart to pump, increasing the work your heart has to do. In addition, animal fats make the blood stickier, increasing the deadly back-and-forth dragging effect on the lining of the arteries.

As outlined in earlier chapters, many factors boost the risk of artery disease, including high blood pressure, high blood fats, age, smoking, sedentary lifestyle, and diabetes. The foods you eat affect all of these risk factors. For example, if you eat foods high in animal fats, you'll have thicker blood. The more you eat, the more you gain, and the less likely you'll feel like jumping on an exercise bike or running a couple of miles to get in shape.

It's clear that a healthy diet is imperative if you want to keep your arteries flexible and free from plaques. I support any healthy diet that's low in animal fat, since this will help lower blood viscosity and lower blood pressure. (I focus on animal fats because, in general, that's where we get large globular molecules of saturated fat, the ones that are solid at room temperature.) If you simply cut out as much animal fat as possible, you'll not only lose weight but feel better too. Your body just doesn't metabolize animal fats very efficiently. Of all the much-touted artery health programs, including this one, the fact remains that only severe calorie reduction has been proved to reverse atherosclerosis.

Obesity and Artery Disease

Despite a tidal wave of exercise videos, diet pills, and low-fat foods, Americans are fatter than ever. A study published in the May 29, 1998, issue of *Science* found that 54 percent of all U.S. adults are overweight—

an increase of about 33 percent since 1978. This obesity rate is one of the highest in the world: about one in three American adults is overweight. All that extra poundage has significant implications for the health of your arteries and your heart.

Obesity has been linked to an increased risk of diabetes, high blood pressure, and elevated blood fats. In fact, obesity in the United States has grown to be such a problem that the American Heart Association (AHA) considers obesity a "major risk factor" for heart disease. This means that obesity carries as much risk to your arteries and heart as smoking, high blood pressure, and a sedentary lifestyle—all factors that you can control if you want to reduce the risk of death and disability from cardiovascular disease. The increased weight means your heart has to pump harder to move the blood through your system (like having to work harder to push a large rock up a hill).

New Weight Standards

Over the years, experts have continually lowered their recommended weight limits, and I totally agree. Keep in mind that a pound of muscle weighs the same as a pound of fat. You may look like Mr. America, but as far as your heart is concerned, you may as well be obese, because it has to work far too hard to pump the blood around your body. Consult Figure 10.1 to find out if you are at a healthy weight.

Muscles do nothing to improve the efficiency of your heart. The heart of a six-foot, 250-pound weight lifter walking up a flight of stairs has to work much harder than that of a six-foot, 160-pound man walking up the same stairs. It's no wonder that the average life expectancy for professional football players is only fifty-five years.

So, don't try to build up your body to get big muscles (lifting weights for strength is very different). In the long run, bulking up is simply not healthy for your arteries.

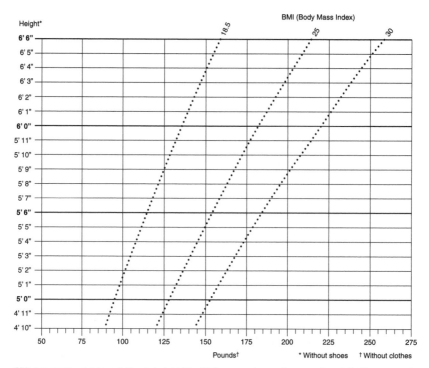

BMI measures weight in relation to height. The BMI ranges shown above are for adults. They are not exact ranges of healthy and unhealthy weights. However, they show that health risk increases at higher levels of overweight and obesity. Even within the healthy BMI range, weight gains can carry health risks for adults.

Directions: Find your weight on the bottom of the graph. Go straight up from that point until you come to the line that matches your height. Then look to find your weight group. Healthy weight—BMI from 18.5 to 25; Overweight—BMI from 25 to 30; Obese—BMI of 30 and above.

Source: Adapted from "Nutrition and Your Health: Dietary Guidelines for Americans." Fifth Edition, 2000. *Home and Garden Bulletin* No. 232. United States Department of Agriculture and United States Department of Health and Human Services.

Figure 10.1   Body Mass Index (BMI) ranges for adults.

Apple or Pear?

If you're too heavy, you're putting your arteries and heart at risk, but *where* you carry your weight is also important, according to data from one new study. The location of fat deposits on your body is controlled genetically; it's inherited from your parents, just like the color of your eyes or hair. Research has found that carrying extra weight around your middle (the so-called apple shape) incurs more health risks than carrying extra weight around hips or thighs ("pear shape"). Overall obesity, however, still puts you at greater risk than storing your fat in the midsection.

In one study, women with the highest waist-to-hip ratios (and a higher waist measurement alone) were significantly more likely to develop heart disease than those with the lowest ratios. Women with a waist measurement of thirty-eight inches or higher had more than three times the risk of developing cardiovascular disease than those with waists of twenty-eight inches or less. A previous study found that abdominal fat is also a risk factor for heart disease in men.

To tell whether or not you're carrying an unhealthy amount of weight around your middle, you can calculate your waist-to-hip ratio (WHR) by dividing your waist measurement by your hip measurement. A healthy WHR for women is less than .85; for men it's less than 1.00.

Americans make eating a ritual: we sit down three times a day and gorge ourselves with too much of the wrong kinds of food. This episodic overloading of the stomach burdens the other organs as well. Instead, don't let yourself get hungry: try grazing. People tend to overeat when they're hungry, waiting until noon to eat just because that's when "lunch" starts, even though they're hungry at 11 A.M. Eating several minimeals and snacks instead is much healthier for your arteries.

Hunger, like thirst, is your body's delayed reaction to deprivation. If you're hungry, you should have eaten an hour ago. Keep fruit, low-fat yogurt, or raisins to munch on during the day. This way, when you do sit down for a meal, you're not famished, and you can better control what you eat and how much.

All of this depressing news about the weight of Americans doesn't bode well for our heart health—but clogged and blocked arteries and weakened hearts aren't inevitable. In fact, losing just 5 percent to 10 percent of your weight can reduce other cardiovascular risk factors such as high blood pressure, diabetes, and elevated blood fats, which, in turn, reduces the thickness of your blood. There are two simple ways to do that: eat fewer calories and animal fats, and exercise. How to get up and get moving in a healthy way is discussed in the next chapter.

If you're going to lose weight, there are plenty of ways you can begin—right now. Nutrition experts will tell you that you don't need to switch overnight from a steady diet of fast food, junk food, and gooey desserts to a strict regimen of grapefruit and water. Instead, begin today by making some simple changes in your diet. The following are some heart-healthy dieting tips from various government sources including the National Heart, Lung, and Blood Institute, the National Center for Research Resources, and the Office of Research on Minority Health:

Do . . .

- Limit meat high in animal fats.
- Trim all visible fat from meat before cooking. Cook in ways that get rid of the fat: broil, bake, stew, roast, poach—do not fry!
- Remove skin from chicken and turkey.
- Use nonstick pans and cooking spray instead of oils and butter.
- Skim off fat from soups.
- Drain off all fat after browning meats.
- Use nonfat milk and low-fat or nonfat sour cream, cottage cheese, and yogurt.
- Double your usual portion of fruits and vegetables, and cut the meat portion in half.
- Drink lots of water.
- Eat smaller portions, several times a day—graze; skip dessert (unless it's fat-free).

Don't . . .

- Eat fried and fast foods.
- Eat organ meats, processed high-fat cold cuts, sausage, or bacon.
- Eat baked goods, snacks, and foods high in saturated fats.
- Drink more than one ounce of alcohol per day.

Your Diet for Life

The Rice Diet . . . the Grapefruit Diet . . . the Steak-and-Water Plan . . . Many of these crash diets focus on weight loss, not on permanent healthful eating, and most experts would agree that these eating plans aren't healthy over the long run. However, health professionals have conflicting opinions about what *does* constitute the best weight-loss diet. What most nutrition experts do agree on is a general plan that includes 30 percent or less of total calories from fat (and not animal fat); no more than 8 percent to 10 percent of total calories from saturated fat; and 2,400 mg or less of sodium per day.

The American Heart Association, the National Heart, Lung, and Blood Institute, the U.S. Department of Agriculture, and the American Dietetic Association all suggest you eat a variety of foods from the six food groups in the food pyramid developed by the Agriculture Department and the Department of Health and Human Services. These organizations recommend that you make most of your selections from the bottom of the pyramid and fewer selections as you work your way up.

What Does the Food Pyramid Mean?

Many consumers are confused by some of the terms in the food pyramid. Specifically, just what *is* a "serving"? Here's a rundown:

- bread: one slice of bread; one-half of a bagel, bun, or English muffin; one ounce (one-half to one cup) ready-to-eat cereal; one-half cup cooked cereal, rice, or pasta (The American Heart Association says starchy vegetables belong in the bread and pasta group; these include potatoes, corn, lima beans, green peas, winter squash, yams, and sweet potatoes.)
- fruit: one medium-size whole fresh fruit; one cup berries or one medium slice of melon; one-half cup chopped, cooked, or canned fruit; one-half cup fruit juice
- vegetables: one cup raw vegetables or one-half cup cooked vegetables; three-quarters cup vegetable juice
- fish, meat, chicken, or beans: two to three ounces cooked fish, poultry, or lean meat; one-half cup cooked dry beans; one-quarter cup tofu; one whole egg or two egg whites; two tablespoons peanut butter, nuts, or seeds (You can eat up to six ounces [cooked] per day of meat, fish, or poultry.)
- dairy: one cup milk or yogurt; one-half cup cottage cheese; 1.5 ounces natural or soy cheese; two ounces processed cheese
- fat: no more than one to two tablespoons a day of canola, safflower, corn, sesame, soybean, sunflower, or olive oil (Avoid coconut oil, palm oil, and hydrogenated fats.)
- sugar: no more than two to two and one-half tablespoons a day

The American Heart Association recommends that for a healthy heart you should eat the following servings per day:

- bread, cereals, pasta, and starchy vegetables: six or more
- vegetables and fruit: five or more
- nonfat milk and low-fat dairy products: two to four
- lean meat, poultry, and seafood: no more than six ounces (weight after cooking)
- fat, oil, nuts, and sweets: sparingly

Oils

Use monounsaturated fats (olive, canola, and peanut oil) for cooking. Studies show that substituting monounsaturated fats for saturated fats such as butter, lard, margarine, and vegetable shortening lowers blood fats and cuts the risk of heart disease, probably by thinning the blood.

Soy

Whether you choose tofu, soy milk, veggie burgers, or other foods made with soy protein, you're protecting your arteries in several ways. The Food and Drug Administration has determined that as little as twenty-five grams of soy protein each day—when combined with a diet that is low in saturated fats and cholesterol—may reduce heart disease. In clinical studies LDL ("bad") cholesterol levels went down in people who ate soy protein. This is good news for your arteries because when cholesterol levels go down, blood viscosity is also reduced. Other clinical studies have shown that soy protein decreases the clumping of blood platelets, which is an early step in forming blood clots.

Whole-Grain Foods

While it's important to get some carbohydrates in your diet, not all carbohydrates are alike. Emphasize whole foods as opposed to highly processed carbohydrates. That means eating brown rice instead of white, choosing whole-grain breads, and avoiding highly processed crackers and chips.

Fiber

Increasing the fiber in your diet may or may not help to reduce the chance of developing heart disease, but it surely can help to keep your bowels regular. Constipation and straining to move your bowels causes enormous spikes in your blood pressure. I don't have a clue as to how fiber reduces the work of the heart in terms of lowering blood pressure or viscosity over the long term, but if it at least keeps you regular, it's worth keeping in your diet.

Try to add more water-soluble fiber (kidney or garbanzo beans, lentils), fruits, and oatmeal. Fiber traps fats and fat by-products in the intestinal tract and keeps them from entering your body. Lima beans, kidney beans, black beans, and other legumes are loaded with soluble fiber. Aim for a bowl of oatmeal in the morning along with a bowl of beans for lunch. (This also helps to ensure regular bowel movements.)

Legumes

Legumes are dry beans and peas, and a heart-healthy choice because they're high in soluble fiber and naturally low in the saturated fat that thickens your blood, according to researchers. Legumes are also a good source of folate, a nutrient known to help lower potentially harmful levels of homocysteine.

Fruits and Vegetables

Aim for five or more medium-size pieces of fruit daily (or half cups of juice). The vitamin C in citrus fruits protects against damage to artery walls, and the phytochemicals in fruit act as antioxidants, fending off damage caused by free radicals that block your arteries. Certain fruits and vegetables are particularly rich in pectin, a soluble fiber that may help thin your blood. Pectin does its job by trapping cholesterol-containing bile acids in the intestine and moving them out of the body. Raisins contain nearly four grams of dietary fiber per one-and-a-half-ounce serving.

Fish: The Way to Go

Eating three to four ounces of fish at least once a week (no more than six ounces a day) can cut your risk of heart disease; the omega-3 fatty acids found in fish help lower cholesterol levels and keep platelets from sticking together and forming unwanted blood clots.

Nuts: Watch Out for the Calories

For a long time, nuts had a bad reputation because of their fat content. Recent studies, though, have found that nuts contain monounsaturated fats and vitamin E which work to lower fat levels. In one new study published in the March 2000 issue of the *Journal of the American Dietetic Association*, researchers found that eating two handfuls of pecans a day lowers blood fat, which will help thin the blood. While three-quarters cup of pecans contains 459 calories and forty-seven grams of fat, twenty-nine of these fat grams are monounsaturated fats, a healthy type of fat that doesn't clog the arteries. Still, those calories add up quickly, so eat nuts in moderation.

Let Them Eat Grapes

If you must have dessert, your best choice is fruit, say experts at the AHA. They also recommend angel food cake, fat-free cookies, graham crackers, gelatin desserts, fat-free frozen yogurt, low-fat ice cream, sherbet, and sorbet. Choose baked snacks instead of fried ones.

Check the Label

Food labels will tell you the total fat, saturated fat, cholesterol, and sodium content of the foods you eat. Labels also list the number of

WHAT DOES THE LABEL MEAN?

Sometimes a label will say that the product is "light" or "low fat." Although these terms and others may sound vague, they actually have specific meanings. Here are the explanations, provided by the National Heart, Lung, and Blood Institute of the National Institutes of Health:

Saturated fat free	Less than ½ gram saturated fat/serving
Low saturated fat	1 gram or less saturated fat/serving
Cholesterol free	Less than 2 milligrams (mg) cholesterol/serving
Low cholesterol	20 mg or less cholesterol/serving
Fat free	Less than ½ gram fat/serving
Low fat	3 grams or less fat/serving
Calorie free	Less than 5 calories/serving
Low calorie	40 calories or less/serving
Sodium free	Less than 5 mg sodium/serving
Low sodium	140 mg or less sodium/serving
Very low sodium	35 mg or less sodium/serving
Light	Half the fat or one-third fewer calories than the regular product
Reduced/less/lower/fewer	Something has been reduced by 25 percent
Lean	Less than 10 grams fat; 4.5 grams or less saturated fat; less than 95 mg cholesterol/serving
Extra lean	Less than 5 grams fat; less than 2 grams saturated fat; less than 95 mg cholesterol/serving

calories in a serving. Look for the heading "Nutrition Facts." Be sure to check the serving size: you may be surprised at how small it is. Then look at the list of ingredients. Limit your intake of products that list any fat or oil first, or that list many fat and oil ingredients.

Vitamins and Supplements

A multivitamin tablet should be on the menu for every person interested in having a healthy heart. A recent study that followed 80,000 women for fourteen years found that the incidence of heart attacks was lowest among those who used multivitamins or who had the highest intake of folic acid and B6 from dietary sources. Also, you should add an iron supplement to your diet if you are menstruating or donating blood on a regular basis.

Folic acid, vitamin B12, and vitamin B6 have all been linked to a possible lower incidence of heart disease and heart attacks. Research suggests that this may be due to the fact that these vitamins lower the levels of the harmful amino acid homocysteine. Of several substances in the blood that are now thought to predict odds for artery disease, the amino acid homocysteine is the one for which the case is strongest. As explained in earlier chapters, it's important to lower homocysteine levels in the blood if you want your arteries to be healthy; dietary supplementation with folic acid can reduce elevated homocysteine levels in most people. The usual therapeutic dose is 1 mg/day and 3 mg of B6.

In a 1995 review of work exploring the relationships among homocysteine levels and artery disease published in the *Journal of the American Medical Association*, researchers proposed that increasing folic acid intake might prevent as many as 50,000 heart attack deaths a year. So, be sure to take a daily multivitamin with 100 percent of the RDA of vitamin B complex and iron.

Fish Oils

Scientists have realized since the early 1970s that artery disease is almost nonexistent among the Eskimos, in spite of their high-calorie, high-fat diet featuring whale meat and oil. Subsequent studies of Eskimo and Japanese populations have proved that fish oil lowers blood viscosity (and/or stickiness) and red blood cell clumping.

While many Eskimos are overweight, with blood fat levels that would normally thicken their blood, fish oil (or more precisely, the omega-3 fatty acids present in the oil) has been shown to lower viscosity by as much as 15 percent in controlled experiments. I believe that the fish oil the Eskimos eat acts as a lubricant; it seems to protect them from artery hardening, injury, and clogging. Studies of the biophysical properties of blood will clarify how and why fish oil is protective.

The omega-3 fatty acids present in fish oils also reduce blood's clotting tendencies, apparently by reducing a chemical involved in clotting called prostaglandin. Some studies have shown that fish oil reduces blood pressure, which would also decrease blood viscosity. Researchers aren't clear on the exact reason why fish oil lowers blood viscosity, only that it does so predictably. That's why I suggest taking a daily fish oil capsule along with your aspirin—right after you brush your teeth in the morning.

Eating fish rich in omega-3 oils is also a good idea. Anchovies and salmon (Atlantic or pink) are the best sources; other varieties have higher omega-3 levels, but they also contain high levels of undesirable fat. (Sardines, for example, also contain twelve grams of fat with the omega-3 fatty acids.)

II

Step Six:
Stay Active

Exercise: it's on everybody's mind. Exercise videos, gyms, equipment—you'd think that with all this attention to exercise, Americans would be the fittest folks on earth. Surprisingly, we're getting heavier even though we're eating less fat than ever before, and experts say it's because more than 60 percent of Americans live sedentary lives.

Regular exercise and physical activity are vital to your physical and emotional health. It conditions and strengthens your heart and makes it work more efficiently. In fact, exercise literally stimulates your body to make more blood vessels that can protect you in case one does close off, especially in the heart.

Exercise can also reduce the risk for diabetes and obesity, two risk factors for atherosclerosis. If you engage in a regular, sustained exercise program, you can prevent or delay the onset of high blood pressure, while lowering the heart's demand for oxygen. This is especially important for people who already have atherosclerosis. However, you must be sure to get your blood pressure down to normal before you begin an exercise program.

Exercise also has other benefits. Regular exercise is an important part of controlling blood sugar levels, losing weight, and reducing the risks of cardiovascular complications for people with diabetes. Many people with leg pain from severe clogged arteries can walk farther without pain after undertaking a regular exercise program.

Exercise Risks

Sounds great, doesn't it? Exercise is vital to artery health—*unless* your blood is too thick, your blood pressure is spiking or too high, or your heart is contracting with too much force.

If any of these situations is true for you, *it's essential for you to get these problems under control* before you begin any type of exercise program. If you start to exercise with any of these conditions, you'll just further injure your arteries with every mile you run or every free weight you lift. If you start to exercise with a heart that's pumping inefficiently, forcing sludge through narrowing arteries, you're just speeding up the artery injury process described in the first two chapters of this book.

This is an error that far too many people make. Ever hear of a seemingly "healthy" athlete who dropped dead in the middle of his daily run? The athlete might have looked healthy on the outside, but odds are, his arteries would have revealed quite a different story: punishingly high blood pressure during exercise, dangerously stiffened arteries, a weakened heart straining to pump sludge through narrowed arteries.

Moreover, heavy physical exertion may sometimes trigger a heart attack, particularly in people who normally lead a sedentary lifestyle, according to a recent Swedish study of 700 men and women who had already had one attack. The heart attack risk was six times higher during strenuous activity than during lighter activity or rest. Still, heavy exertion only rarely triggers heart attacks, accounting for about 6 percent of those in people aged forty-five to seventy. Those at highest risk said they had exercised "very little" throughout their lives or had rarely performed the strenuous tasks that triggered their attacks.

The bottom line is that you should start slow but keep doing something on a regular basis—for life. Previous research, including a U.S. study of more than 1,200 heart attack patients, found that the risk for an exertion-triggered heart attack steadily declines the more a person exercises.

Before Starting a Program

You can't tell whether it's safe to start an exercise program just by looking in the mirror. You can be an energetic thirty-something with a physique like Charles Atlas and still have the arteries of an eighty-year-old. (Remember that tennis great Arthur Ashe had heart bypass surgery in his early thirties.) To find out if it's safe to exercise, you need to go to your doctor for a complete physical (see Chapter 5). In fact, the U.S. surgeon general advises every man over age forty and woman over age fifty to consult a doctor before beginning a vigorous physical activity program.

You need to know what your blood pressure is doing while you're exercising, not just while you're peacefully sitting there in the doctor's office leafing through *People* magazine. The only way to tell what happens to your blood pressure while exercising is to have an exercise stress test, which measures your blood pressure while you're active. Some people may have a totally normal resting blood pressure that spikes to fearsome levels during exercise, but you won't know if you're one of them unless a cardiologist gives you a stress test.

Get Started!

Being a couch potato increases the risk of heart disease by contributing directly to heart-related problems and increasing the chances of developing other risk factors, such as high blood pressure and diabetes. It's a problem that's getting worse in this country, especially among women. According to the first-ever *Surgeon General's Report on Physical Activity and Health*, 60 percent of American women don't get the recommended amount of physical activity, while more than 25 percent aren't active at all.

Fortunately, being "physically active" doesn't mean you have to participate in the Ironman Triathlon. The surgeon general's report and other research conclude that as little as 30 minutes of moderate activity on most (preferably all) days of the week helps protect artery health. Tooling around on your bike, raking up that pile of leaves in the backyard, plunking in a bunch of petunias in the garden, or walking around the block will help. Whatever you do, do something every day that you can do for the *rest of your life*.

You can divide the thirty-minute activity into shorter periods of at least ten minutes each and still get the health benefits, according to the National Heart, Lung, and Blood Institute. In fact, two recent studies indicate that moderate daily physical activity (such as taking the stairs instead of the elevator) is as effective as a structured exercise program in improving heart function, lowering blood pressure, and maintaining or losing weight.

If you want to make exercise a part of your life, you'd better choose something you like, or it just won't happen. Fortunately, it doesn't take hours of painful, sweat-soaked exertion to achieve most of these health benefits. Too many people think that an exercise program means you need to work out as if you were training for the Olympics. It's not true.

How to Exercise

You'll be more likely to stay with your program if you choose activities you like. Try to do some type of activity every day, or at least three days a week. Start out slowly, and gradually build up your exercise time and frequency; a little goes a long way. For example, formerly inactive people who take a brisk thirty-minute walk each day will be able to lower their heart attack risk more than will joggers who boost their regimens from three runs a week to five. As further evidence, a 1996 preliminary report from the Nurses Health Study noted that women who walked briskly at least three hours a week had a 54 percent lower risk of heart attack and stroke than those who were inactive.

But no exercise program will work unless you actually do it. Again, the main thing is to find a program that works for you and that you can continue for the rest of your life. Many Americans have an "all-or-nothing" attitude toward exercise: if they can't spend thirty minutes three times a week on a program, they don't bother to exercise at all. But the fact is that any activity you choose is better than nothing.

If you're having trouble starting at all, start small:

- Park farther from your destination and walk the extra distance.
- If you take a bus to work, get off a stop earlier and walk.
- Take the stairs instead of the elevator.
- Get off the elevator one floor before your destination and walk the remaining flight.
- Walk, don't drive, to do your errands.
- Use the bathroom one floor up or down from your office.

After you get your blood pressure and viscosity under control and you feel that moderate exercise is no longer enough, you can move

EXERCISE CALORIES BURNED PER HOUR

Exercise is a good way to burn calories. Here is a brief list of exercises and the number of calories associated with a one-hour workout for a 150-pound person:

Cycling 6 mph	240
Walking 2 mph	240
Walking 3 mph	320
Tennis (singles)	400
Jogging 7 mph	920
Cross-country skiing	700
Swimming 25 yards per minute	275

into a more vigorous heart and lung conditioning program. But remember: you need a program that works for you for the rest of your life, such as:

- brisk, sustained walking
- skating
- jumping rope
- aerobic dancing or water aerobics
- hiking
- rowing
- swimming
- biking (stationary or bicycle)
- cross-country skiing
- jogging
- squash or tennis
- basketball
- golf
- stair climbing

How Long?

You should exercise within your *target heart rate range* for at least thirty minutes each session, according to the American College of Sports Medicine. It's best to maintain your training intensity for at least thirty consecutive minutes.

Formal Program

Many people find that a formal exercise program can be helpful. Also, exercising in a group can make it easier and more fun. This usually involves setting aside a period of time, at least several times a week, to deliberately focus on increasing fitness. A complete fitness program combines activities to improve flexibility, strength, and endurance. Vigorous exercises can improve the fitness of your heart, which can lower heart disease risk. These types of aerobic activity include jogging, swimming, and jumping rope. Walking, biking, and dancing can

HOW TO CALCULATE TARGET HEART RATE RANGE

To calculate your target heart rate range during exercise on your own:

1. Calculate your *maximum* heart rate by subtracting your age from 220.
2. Multiply this maximum by 60 percent.
3. Multiply this maximum by 80 percent.
4. This is your target heart rate range.

Example: A forty-year-old man would have a maximum heart rate of 180 beats per minute. To exercise at training level, he must keep his heart rate between 108 beats (60 percent of maximum) and 144 beats (80 percent of maximum) per minute.

also strengthen the heart if you do them briskly for at least thirty minutes, three or four times a week. If you're weak or frail, you should start slowly; begin with stretching and strength training, and add aerobics later.

Each exercise session should start with a stretching period of about five minutes to give your body a chance to warm up. After the aerobic exercise or vigorous conditioning period, take another five minutes to cool down with a slower exercise pace.

Some Discomfort Is Normal

If you haven't exercised recently, you may experience some discomfort in the beginning. It's natural to feel your heart beat faster, your breathing speed up, and your body get warmer during aerobic exercise. It's normal as well to feel muscle and joint tenderness during the early weeks of training, and to be a little more tired in the evenings. You'll also sleep better. You didn't get out of shape overnight—you won't get back into shape overnight. Be patient with yourself, but beyond a wholesome discipline, be kind to yourself.

What's *Not* Normal

If you have a heart condition, your doctor may suggest that you engage in a monitored exercise program at first. The American Heart Association advises you to stop exercising until you have talked to your doctor if you have any of the following symptoms while exercising:

- nausea
- dizziness

- excessive shortness of breath
- fainting
- discomfort in your upper body, chest, arm, neck, or jaw
- bone or joint pain during or after exercise

Be aware of activities that may put excess strain on joints. You need them to last as well.

12

The alarm never went off. Your best suit is lying in a wrinkled pile in the closet, and your good shoes need to be polished. At breakfast, your son suddenly remembers he needs a Mexican sombrero for the school play this afternoon. The cat throws up on the carpet, the dishwasher is making that funny noise again, and as you run for the car, you remember you forgot to fill the tank and the gauge is on "E." It's not even 7 A.M., and already you feel that vein in your temple start to throb . . .

How many of your mornings start this way? If you're like most Americans, stress has pretty much become a way of life. But when you get so stressed that you feel as if you might explode, you can bet it's having a negative effect on your heart—starting with your arteries. Stress is a pervasive health problem in our culture. In fact, one out of every five people responds to stress in a destructive way.

Health experts know that for some people, stress, anger, and hostility contribute to thickened blood and high blood pressure, increasing the risk of atherosclerosis and heart disease. Scientists don't know exactly how stress plays its deadly role, but I suspect that someday we will find that the brain is the ultimate master of how fast our arteries age.

We don't know as much about how stress affects the arteries as we do about other risk factors, such as smoking, high blood pressure, family history, diabetes, diet, obesity, and physical inactivity. And we still don't know whether stress acts as an independent risk, or whether it merely aggravates the other risk factors you've already got.

The "Fight-or-Flight" Response

No matter how you define *stress*—as a type of situation that triggers symptoms, as the changes in your body that result, or as the symptoms you feel—health experts agree that stress has been essential for human survival. There is a real need for humans to be able to respond quickly to danger; your body's response to stress exists as a vestige of the "fight-or-flight" response that ensured the survival of our species.

When you perceive or anticipate a threatening or stressful situation, part of your nervous system releases stress hormones to prepare you to react: to run away from danger, or to fight if you can't run. These hormones are pumped throughout the body to speed up breathing, increase heartbeat, and tense muscles. The sympathetic nervous system raises your blood pressure. It directs blood flow less to your fingers, skin, and toes and more to the large muscles in your arms and legs, where it's needed for action.

Recent research has focused on both the protective and damaging effect of your body's hormonal response to stress. When secreted in response to acute stress, stress hormones protect and help you adapt to the stress. But when stress hormones are not turned off, overexposure to these hormones may injure your arteries. You probably don't even realize how many inconsequential stresses you deal with every day, but each one probably takes a toll on your body. If you're under constant stress, these hormones may never drop below crisis levels.

Stress and Your Body

Years of repeated stresses can lead to an array of health problems, according to a review article of more than 100 stress studies in the January 15, 1999, issue of the *New England Journal of Medicine.* Whether it's the stress of daily life, the pressures of an executive job, frustrations of a lower-level position, or even social upheaval in an unstable country, the chronic activation of the body's stress-response systems can damage your heart and your health. As adrenaline, released by stress, pours into your bloodstream, it increases the contraction of the heart and raises blood pressure, and in one way or another, it increases blood viscosity.

Investigators at the University of Pittsburgh have found an association between mental stress and atherosclerosis, according to findings published in the December 2, 1999, issue of *Circulation.* They suggest that bursts of high blood pressure in response to stress may injure the inner linings of blood vessels. Researchers found that patients who responded to stress with the highest blood pressure spikes showed thicker carotid artery walls.

The link between artery wall thickness and high blood pressure response to stress did not depend on other conditions such as resting blood pressure, risk factors for heart disease, and the existence of heart disease. Even among men younger than fifty-five who had no symptoms of heart disease and who took no medications, investigators found a significant link between exaggerated blood pressure responses to stress and thickened artery walls.

Studies also show that job stress can chronically raise blood pressure—and that stress due to lack of control on the job increases the risk of coronary heart disease. One study of stress resulting from social instability showed that cardiovascular disease largely accounted for a nearly 40 percent jump in the death rate among Russian men following the fall of communism.

Emotions and Your Heart

In the past, health experts thought of people prone to heart attacks as pressured and driven. Research linking anger to heart problems goes back to at least the 1960s, when California cardiologists Meyer Friedman and Ray Rosenman coined the term *type A* to describe edgy, impatient people who were more likely to have heart attacks.

Today, experts believe that the people at biggest risk are those who experience negative emotions such as depression, anger, and hostility (all of which create stress). In Norway, for example, studies found that patients with congestive heart failure who also suffered from severe depression were four times more likely to die within two years of treatment than patients who weren't depressed. And researchers at Johns Hopkins Medical School found that men who reported having at least one bout of clinical depression were more than twice as likely as others to later develop coronary heart disease or have a heart attack. In some cases, the heart attack didn't occur until ten years after the depression set in.

Certain chronic emotional responses to stress, such as hostility, aggression, and cynicism, also have been associated with atherosclerosis. If you're chronically hostile or cynical, your body is more likely to react to stress with larger increases in heart rate, blood pressure, and stress hormones than people with less hostile feelings. This isn't good for your arteries, your heart, or your general health.

Serotonin, a brain chemical that affects mood and personality, may be the link between stress and heart problems. Among people who have a biological tendency toward negative moods, stress appears to trigger a response as if the body were experiencing an actual physical injury. In fact, research clearly shows that stress and many psychological symptoms appear to be directly related to viscosity—so that the more stress you feel, the thicker your blood tends to be.

What You Can Do

Luckily, the stressful events in your life and your behavioral reactions are uniquely yours. You can learn to modify your appraisal of potentially stressful situations and how you deal with them. You can even exert some control over your physical reactions, which can help you lead a healthier, more balanced life. The key is to take action today. Reducing stress is an excellent way to prevent and treat atherosclerosis.

The first step to managing your stress is to identify it. Many people underestimate the amount of stress they encounter in their daily lives. To figure out the stress burden you're struggling with, you must recognize what sort of stress you encounter every day.

In a now-famous 1967 study, Drs. Thomas H. Holmes and Richard H. Rahe created a do-it-yourself stress test called the Social Readjustment Rating Scale, first published in the *Journal of Psychosomatic Research*. With this self-test, they examined the stress (measured as "life changes") of experiences ranging from the death of a partner to a traffic ticket. Part of the premise is that *any* change usually brings about stress, even if it's something fun like going to the beach on vacation. Their scale is adapted here.

To find out what stress you're experiencing, check all of the following life changes that apply to you over the past year, and add up the points, then see where you fall:

Death of a partner	100
Divorce	73
Marital separation	65
Jail term	63
Death of a close family member	63
Personal injury or illness	53
Marriage	50

Fired from job	47
Marital reconciliation	45
Retirement	45
Change in family member's health	44
Pregnancy	40
Sex problems	39
New family member	39
New business	39
Change in financial status	38
Death of a close friend	37
Different line of work	36
More arguments with partner	35
Mortgage or loan	31
Foreclosure	30
Change in job responsibility	29
Child leaves home	29
In-law trouble	29
Outstanding personal achievement	28
Partner starts or stops work	26
Begin or end school	26
Change in living conditions	25
Trouble with boss	23
Change in work hours	20
Change in residence	20
Change in school	20
Change in recreation	19
Change in church activities	19
Change in sleeping habits	16
Change in number of family get-togethers	15
Change in eating habits	15
Vacation	13

Holiday celebration   12
Minor violation of law   11

POINTS

300+	Your stress level is high. You need stress-intervention techniques now!
150–299	Borderline high stress. Reduce the number of high-impact changes in your life, if possible, and learn stress-reduction techniques.
0–149	Low stress level.

Symptoms of Stress

Sometimes it's obvious when you're feeling stressed, but at other times your symptoms may be so subtle that you don't even recognize your situation. Common symptoms of stress include:

- headaches (migraine or tension)
- back, neck, and shoulder aches
- tiredness
- fingernail biting or nervous tics
- sleeplessness
- restlessness
- lowered sex drive
- stomach problems (acid, gas, diarrhea, constipation)
- shallow breathing or sighing
- teeth grinding or jaw clenching
- sweaty or cold hands
- excess perspiration
- forgetfulness, distraction
- pessimism

- indecision or inefficiency
- cynicism or hostility
- poor self-esteem or morale
- frustration, anxiety, depression, boredom
- anger, resentfulness, apathy, irritability
- substance abuse
- withdrawal or disorganization
- increased number of accidents

How to Cope with Stress

Once you recognize the symptoms of stress, you can develop more effective coping skills. Fortunately, there are many simple things you can do right now to help manage stress in your life that don't cost anything.

Following is a list of coping responses suggested by the American Heart Association:

- Listen to music; watch TV or movies; read.
- Get more sleep. Fatigue is a common underlying factor exacerbating most stress in our lives.
- Write a journal.
- Distract yourself: attend a play, lecture, or symphony.
- Exercise: play sports, run, stretch, lift weights.
- Relax: pray, meditate, or do yoga; try a massage; take a warm bath, shower, or hot tub.
- Engage in a hobby.
- Get fresh air: force yourself to go outdoors, enjoy nature.
- Laugh. Humor can be a powerful antidote. Read a funny book or rent a classic comedy video.

- Escape: get away on a vacation, take a trip, or go camping.
- Seek support: talk things over with friends, listen to relaxation tapes, read self-help books.

Stress-Reduction Techniques

All of the foregoing suggestions are things you can do right away, without any training or support from a health professional. It's often helpful to seek other, more formal methods of stress reduction as well; if you use a combination of approaches, you increase your chance of successfully managing stress. This is effective both in preventing atherosclerosis and in healing after a person has been diagnosed with heart disease.

In fact, heart disease patients who learn how to manage their stress with relaxation and biofeedback are 77 percent less likely to have a heart attack or require cardiac surgery than patients who receive only standard medical care, according to a study published in the October 27, 1999, *Archives of Internal Medicine.* Unfortunately, few heart patients receive stress management in any form; only 10 percent of patients who would benefit from rehabilitation services participate in such programs.

Here's what you should investigate if you're interested in reducing your stress:

- progressive muscle relaxation
- breathing exercises
- meditation
- biofeedback-assisted relaxation
- cognitive and behavior therapy
- antistress drugs

Progressive Muscle Relaxation

If you practice relaxation techniques such as muscle relaxation, deep breathing, and meditation, you're less likely to suffer from certain types of heart disease or a fatal heart attack. If you have undergone heart surgery, you can use these techniques to help you relax your body and enhance your recovery. This type of general relaxation is easy to learn.

The American Heart Association suggests the following technique:

1. Get into a comfortable position, with your head and neck supported.
2. Close your eyes and tense each muscle group.
3. Keep the muscles tense for a few seconds as you continue to breathe, then slowly relax the muscles of your hands and arms, face, neck and shoulders, stomach and abdomen, buttocks and thighs, calves, and toes.
4. Then sit quietly for several minutes and enjoy the feeling of a relaxed body before you slowly open your eyes.

Yoga is another good way to relax. Take a yoga class and practice by yourself at home. Yoga can relax tense muscles, teach you better breathing, lower your blood pressure, decrease your heart rate, and divert your mind from stress.

Breathing and Stress

Most of us don't breathe correctly—from the diaphragm, the way trained singers do. Deep breathing is essential for stress management. Of all the things you can do to ease anxiety and stress, forming healthy breathing habits can produce the most dramatic results. When you become stressed, you start taking shallow breaths.

Whole books have been written about how to do relaxation breathing; check them out if you're interested. Meanwhile, here's a quick stress-buster technique:

1. Sit in a chair with feet flat, thighs parallel to the floor.
2. Inhale through your nose and breathe deeply, without forcing. *Let your abdomen expand.* Place your hand on your abdomen, and slowly push the air out.
3. In one continuous breath, fill your lungs with air. Feel your chest expand fully and your shoulders rise.
4. Exhale slowly through your nose. Breathing out should take longer than breathing in.
5. Do this for at least one minute. Don't strain. Concentrate on keeping your breathing deep.

Meditation, Stress, and Heart Disease

Meditation may help reduce atherosclerosis and risk of heart attack and stroke, according to findings published in *Stroke,* a journal of the American Heart Association. Studies have found that people who meditate exhibited a decrease of 0.098 millimeter in artery wall thickness; the control group had an increase of 0.054 millimeter. Researchers say that these and other findings suggest that the distinct state of restful alertness during meditation may trigger self-repair mechanisms in the body, which lead to the improvement of atherosclerosis. Other studies have shown that reducing stress by meditating lowered blood pressure in people with high levels of stress and multiple risk factors for high blood pressure.

Biofeedback

You can also reduce stress through biofeedback, identifying the sources of stress and controlling your physical and mental responses. Biofeedback systems use an electronic sensor to measure stress in your body. The machine measures an unconscious activity (blood pressure, pulse, body temperature, muscle tension, and so on). As you practice some version of relaxation, you get feedback about your body from the machine. After some practice, you can learn to associate how you feel with your internal body process. For example, you get to know how it feels when your blood pressure rises or falls. After even more practice (you need to be dedicated!), you can learn to lower your blood pressure or slow your heart rate by using a variety of techniques.

You should learn the proper technique from a professional at a hospital or university program. You can then buy a device to measure your own blood pressure and continue the biofeedback at home.

Cognitive/Behavioral Therapy

Your doctor may suggest psychotherapy to pinpoint stressful events or conditions, and to help you learn how to reduce stress. You may think of stress as something that happens *to* you, but how you approach your life—your thoughts and your attitudes—can have a major impact on your stress level. When your attitude is negative or hostile, you can experience much more stress.

Behavioral or cognitive therapy, provided by a trained professional, can help you discern how your thoughts and behavior affect your stress level. The therapist can then help you learn tools to change those thoughts or behaviors, which will lower your stress. Group therapy is often valuable for people who share a stressful life situation.

Antistress Drugs

If none of the previous suggestions work, your doctor may suggest an antistress drug such as Valium (diazepam) or Xanax (alprazolam). These can be especially effective if you have symptoms of stress from a specific event, such as a death in the family. However, tranquilizers should be used only for a short time because they are habit-forming. Alternatively, your doctor may suggest an antidepressant for stress and anxiety, such as one of the many new and highly effective selective serotonin reuptake inhibitors (SSRIs).

Part 3

Special Populations

13

Children and Atherosclerosis

Jim's favorite meal is a Big Mac, a Super Size Fry, and a Super Size soda. He spends his free time sprawled on the couch nibbling on potato chips, clutching his TV remote, and playing video games instead of kicking around a soccer ball or riding a bike. Jim doesn't know it, but his blood pressure has already started to rise. Streaks of fatty deposits are beginning to appear along the walls of his arteries. At the age of twelve, Jim's arteries already look as if they belong to a forty-year-old man.

Most people think that high blood pressure and clogged, thickened arteries are conditions of age. We picture middle-aged men and women eating too much rich food, smoking and drinking to excess, and not getting enough exercise.

That's certainly part of the picture. But middle-aged people don't go to bed one night healthy and wake up with atherosclerosis; the whole gradual process begins much, much earlier. In fact, mounting research has shown that for many people, high blood pressure and atherosclerosis has its roots in early childhood.

American children today make up one of the largest at-risk groups for developing heart disease. The President's Council on Physical Fitness and Sports says that 40 percent of children ages five to eight exhibit at least one risk factor for atherosclerosis: high blood pressure, high blood cholesterol, or low capacity for exertion. Other risk factors such as obesity and cigarette smoking have also been shown to contribute to the development of atherosclerosis regardless of a person's age.

It's not just boys who are at risk. New research shows that girls as young as fifteen develop streaks of fat on the walls of their arteries, and some have as many fat deposits as men three times their age. At first, these fat streaks aren't a threat to young girls' health, but the streaks are an indication that the artery is beginning to stiffen, which paves the way for the creation of plaque, the thick fatty deposits that can clog arteries and cause a heart attack later.

Fortunately, most women are protected from heart disease in their youth despite these early fat deposits because of their monthly menstrual periods, which keeps their blood thin. As long as women menstruate, their blood viscosity is much lower than that of men.

There's one exception to this premenopausal protection: it doesn't work if a teenage girl smokes. Even if she's still menstruating, she will dramatically increase her chances of artery disease because smoking will cause her blood to be stickier and thicker than it should be. And as noted in Chapter 8, that's one of the primary risk factors for developing atherosclerosis. This problem is magnified if these women are taking birth control pills.

High Blood Pressure

The problem of atherosclerosis begins with high blood pressure. Even so, for a long time, pediatricians didn't bother to measure the blood pressure of their young patients, since it never occurred to anyone that high blood pressure was a problem in very young people.

But today, we know that children as young as two can have high blood pressure—usually related to being overweight. In fact, one recent study of youngsters aged two to five revealed that about 10 percent had borderline high blood pressure.

Because of these alarming findings, the American Heart Association and the American Academy of Pediatrics state that all children should have their blood pressure measured each year beginning at age three in order to detect the presence of atherosclerosis and heart disease as early as possible.

If your family has a history of early heart disease or high cholesterol (which suggests that the blood may be too viscous), it's important to have your child's cholesterol levels checked yearly and watched for increases. Once the blood viscosity test is available, you should do a yearly check on this as well.

Atherosclerosis in Children

Since high blood pressure ultimately leads to atherosclerosis, it's no surprise that studies have found it's also fairly common for American children to have partially blocked arteries. By age twelve, as many as 70 percent of children have fatty deposits in their arteries, a problem that only gets significantly worse as the child gets older. According to studies at the Cleveland Clinic Foundation, evidence of atherosclerosis in supposedly healthy donated hearts was found even among teenagers. Five of thirty-two donors under the age of twenty showed early signs of atherosclerosis.

It is also not surprising that the more risk factors a child has—family history, obesity, smoking, thickened blood, high blood pressure—the more fatty deposits there are, and here again, the buildup only gets worse with age. Since about 42 percent of the people discharged from hospitals for coronary heart disease are under sixty-five, many of these adults have children who may have coronary heart disease risk factors that need attention.

Lack of Exercise

It's a sad fact of American life today: far too many of our children spend most of their time hunched over a computer or lying on a couch, watching TV or playing video games. Experts estimate that about half of all American children don't get enough exercise.

Since obesity is the risk factor most strongly correlated with high blood pressure and atherosclerosis, it's truly alarming that more than 25 percent of the nation's children are overweight or obese, according to researchers at the University of Colorado Health Science Center in Denver. One of the primary causes of obesity is not getting enough exercise. The other is poor diet.

"Addiction" to Fat

Of course, diet is inextricably linked to high blood pressure, blood viscosity, and atherosclerosis. My suggestion: keep only healthy foods in the house. *If it's not in the house, they can't eat it.* Don't buy chips, cookies, or soda. Stick to fruit, vegetables, and other heart-healthy foods.

The diet of America's children is often appalling. In one study, more than 80 percent of high school students ate diets that exceeded the recommended levels of total fat and saturated fat. More than a third had elevated levels of LDL cholesterol and low levels of HDL cholesterol, which suggests they also have thick blood. Ten percent had blood pressure higher than normal. The students' weight was directly linked to high blood pressure and the buildup of fatty deposits in the carotid artery.

The effects of a poor diet include more than only high blood pressure and high blood viscosity in adolescence; the evidence of heart disease by this age can already be seen on ultrasound examination. Dr. Albert Sanchez and colleagues at the Pacific Health Education Center in Bakersfield, California, asked 211 students from three high schools about their lifestyles and eating habits. The researchers also measured blood pressure, height, and weight and took blood to measure blood fat and uric acid levels. Finally, researchers measured the thickness of the students' carotid artery walls using ultrasound.

They discovered that students who ate low-fat, high-vegetable diets had thinner, healthier artery walls; students who consumed more fat had thicker artery walls. The more junk food a teenager ate, the thicker the artery walls became. In fact, the ultrasound pictures were so dramatic that many students who saw the graphic evidence of their unhealthy arteries immediately began to improve their poor diets.

There is no doubt about it. Science has proved that eating animal fats kills.

Smoking Compounds the Problem

If a quarter of our children are on their way to early atherosclerosis, the last thing we'd want to see is a cigarette habit added to the risk factors. Yet, while smoking today is certainly declining in popularity among adults, there are still about 9 million children who live with at least one smoker and are exposed to secondhand smoke every day of their lives. Even more sobering is the fact that every day, 3,000 young people in this country become smokers.

Keeping Kids Healthy

Most parents can't imagine not giving their children polio vaccines. Likewise, we wouldn't send kids off to football camp without the proper safety gear, or allow them to go to school without their homework completed. But when it comes to teaching kids a healthy lifestyle—and modeling one ourselves—many of us fall woefully short.

Given that so many children are at risk for atherosclerosis, it's imperative that we teach our children how to make healthy choices, especially in families with a history of atherosclerosis, obesity, diabetes, heart disease, or stroke.

Because American children today don't usually get enough physical activity and eat too much fatty food, parents need to help develop a family exercise routine and introduce children to better eating patterns. You can set a good example by pursuing a healthy lifestyle yourself.

Since eating patterns and habits are developed early in life, it makes sense to teach children to eat a healthy diet. Children should be offered a wide variety of food to obtain as many vitamins and minerals as possible from their diet, in addition to a daily multivitamin. If there is a history of heart disease in your family, it's a good idea to model healthy eating habits by following a low-fat, high-fiber diet.

Here are a few ways you and your family can thin your blood by healthy eating:

- Teach children to eat by "grazing."
- Encourage children to eat more fish.
- Have your kids eat low-fat and fat-free dairy products, such as child-size yogurt or reduced-fat string cheese.
- Prepare at least one vegetarian meal per week, such as spaghetti with meatless sauce or tortillas with fat-free refried beans mixed with vegetables.
- Serve fresh fruit for snacks or dessert.

CHILDREN UNDER AGE TWO

The American Academy of Pediatrics advises that parents should not restrict fats for youngsters under age two, since infants and toddlers need more calories and fat for the proper development of the brain and nervous system. After age two, you can introduce the same healthy diet you choose for yourself.

- Serve high-fiber cereal without added sugar, together with low-fat milk. (Most cereal now contains additional folate, which appears to decrease risk of cardiovascular disease.)
- Cut out animal fats.
- Don't buy junk food.

In order to slow the progression of atherosclerosis, the American Heart Association recommends that most children *over age two* eat whole grains, fruits and vegetables, and nonfat dairy products, with no more than 30 percent of calories from fat and less than 10 percent from saturated fat. Allow your child to graze—if she's hungry, let her eat. Don't force large meals on children. Trying to get them in the habit of eating three large meals a day is a bad idea.

Serving Suggestions

There are a few things to keep in mind if you want to serve healthy meals (nothing fried!) to your children, according to the American Heart Association. Be sure to serve breakfast—but hold the greasy fried eggs, bacon, and sausage, and cut back or eliminate butter, cream, doughnuts, coffee cakes, and cookies.

Instead, try offering whole-wheat toast, low-fat cottage cheese, and fresh fruit. Scramble the whites of the eggs only. Use fresh fruit or raisins to sweeten oatmeal or other whole-grain cereals. Whole-grain waffles can make a good alternative.

Pack lunches with rice cakes, pita pockets, or whole-wheat or corn tortillas. Instead of using high-fat luncheon meats, pack sliced chicken or turkey, or chicken salad with low-fat mayonnaise. Go easy on the peanut butter (it may be a good source of protein, but also has a lot of fat); combine it with raisins, dates, or bananas instead of sugar-loaded jelly. Add low-fat yogurt, fresh fruits and vegetables, low-salt pretzels, and low-fat cookies.

For dinner, choose lean cuts of red meat (no more than twice a week), lean poultry and fish (no fatty sauce!); fresh vegetables, grains, rice, beans, pasta without high-fat cheeses and butter, nonfat milk or fruit juice, and low-fat desserts or fresh fruits. While you're at it, try to sit down as a family when you eat. Studies have found that family-style meals tend to provide more nutrients and better balance and variety than meals eaten alone. The more often a child eats dinner with the family, the healthier the eating patterns appear to be.

Early Education

It's never too early to begin efforts to keep the blood thin and help prevent heart disease and stroke, before bad habits develop. We should teach our children:

- the dangers of smoking and alcohol
- nutritious eating habits
- an active lifestyle
- the benefits of exercise
- the benefits of daily vitamins and fish oil
- grazing

14

Diabetes and Atherosclerosis

If you've got diabetes, you need to know that you're also at much higher risk for developing atherosclerosis. High blood pressure and high blood viscosity are two of the most important links with both atherosclerosis and diabetes.

There are two types of diabetes, and both can lead to atherosclerosis. Type I is the more serious and usually requires people to take insulin. Type II often occurs in middle age and is known as "adult onset diabetes"; it can often be controlled by diet alone.

People with type I diabetes don't produce insulin. Insulin is the hormone that helps blood sugar move into the body's cells; without it, the body can't control blood sugar. If left uncontrolled, high blood sugar levels lead to thicker blood. Usually appearing in early life, this type of diabetes is fairly rare (it accounts for less than 5 percent of diabetes cases), but it can have a great impact on a patient's life.

In type II diabetes, the body's cells become resistant to insulin, and the pancreas can't produce enough to overcome that resistance. Type II diabetes is the more common form; both obesity and lack of exercise contribute to insulin resistance and can lead to diabetes.

High Blood Pressure

The beginning of the book documented how high blood pressure and thickened, viscous blood can lead to atherosclerosis. Diabetes, high blood pressure, and high blood viscosity are all interrelated.

When the body fails to respond to normal insulin levels, insulin production increases—but high levels of insulin raise blood pressure and encourage the fat deposits in artery walls. The result: clogged coronary arteries. In fact, high blood pressure and high blood viscosity are about twice as common in people with diabetes.

High Blood Viscosity

People who have diabetes also tend to have thickened blood. When the diabetes is in poor control and sugar spills into the bloodstream, the red blood cells become less flexible, getting stickier and clumping more easily. Platelets, another blood component, also stick together more in people who have developed diabetes—even in the early stages of the disease. This is why low-dose aspirin therapy is recommended by the American Diabetes Association. (It's also recommended for people who smoke, have high blood pressure, have a family history of atherosclerosis, are overweight, or have high lipid levels; see Chapter 7.)

Diabetes Complications

Unfortunately, atherosclerosis isn't the only complication of diabetes. Leg problems and blindness because of poor circulation are also common.

Diabetes is the number one cause of blindness in the United States today. While the reason for this is still unknown, I believe it's due to the fact that capillaries supplying blood to the back of the eye have adapted to the injury they incur from deformed red blood cells. As these inflexible red blood cells are pushed through capillaries, they scour the lining of the capillaries like little Brillo pads; in response, the capillaries adapt to the injury by closing themselves off, causing blindness. The same happens to the kidneys and feet, places most dependent on capillaries to survive.

What You Can Do

If you have diabetes, there are lots of things you can do to lessen the risk of developing atherosclerosis. These include:

- Control blood viscosity by the seven-step plan described in this book.
- Donate blood.
- Stop smoking—a *must.*
- Treat high blood pressure.

Control Your Weight

Weight loss can decrease the demand for insulin, and exercise can help you to use up excess blood glucose, which can prevent (or at least slow down) the onset of diabetes. A low-fat, low-cholesterol diet can decrease blood lipid levels. Losing weight also can help you lower blood pressure. In addition, it's important to get regular aerobic exercise to help you lose weight and boost your overall cardiovascular health.

Take It Personally

People with diabetes should work with a dietitian to personalize a healthy eating plan. Basically, however, what's healthy for a person with diabetes is what's healthy for anyone else: less fat, fewer sugary foods, and a variety of fresh vegetables, fruits, lean meat, and fish.

People with type I diabetes need to be obsessively careful about planning meals to coincide with the time when insulin is working the hardest; monitoring blood sugar levels is extremely important. Attention to meals should help avoid low blood sugar.

People with type II diabetes can often manage their condition with diet alone, aiming for healthy weight, lower levels of blood fats, normal blood pressure, and control of blood sugar.

Women and Diabetes

It's been shown dramatically that women have a much higher risk of diabetes—and subsequent atherosclerosis. All other things being equal, if you're a woman with diabetes, you have five times the risk of heart disease; men with diabetes have twice the risk.

Women with type II diabetes tend to carry more weight around the abdomen, have lower HDL cholesterol, and have higher blood pressure—all of which may increase their risk of developing cardiovascular disease, according to data from more than 4,500 Native Americans enrolled in the Strong Heart Study. Unfortunately, while certain risk factors for atherosclerosis (cigarette smoking, high blood fats, and high blood pressure) seem to be declining, type II diabetes is increasing.

Control of blood sugar can be vital to artery health. People diagnosed with type I diabetes after age thirty have a high risk for heart disease if their blood sugar control is poor. In one new study of 177 people with type I diabetes who were followed for up to seven years, the risk of dying from heart disease was seven times higher among people who didn't adequately control their blood sugar levels. Those with poor blood sugar control had a three times higher risk for death or nonfatal heart attacks than those with better sugar control. This is why strict blood sugar control is important for every person with diabetes who wants to avoid all complications.

If You Suspect Diabetes

If you're at risk for atherosclerosis, it's important that your doctor check you for diabetes, because some symptoms (slow-healing infections, tingling or numbness in the hands and feet, blurred vision) may not appear at first.

The American Diabetes Association recommends routine screening for everyone at age forty-five, using one of the following tests:

- Fasting blood glucose: A blood sample is tested for sugar after you've stopped eating for between ten and sixteen hours. A measure of 126 mg/dL (milligrams per deciliter) or higher indicates diabetes. (Results are confirmed with a repeat test on a different day.)
- Nonfasting blood glucose: This blood test can be taken anytime, whether you've eaten or not. A reading above 200 mg/dL would confirm diabetes if the results are the same on a different day.
- Glucose tolerance test: After an initial blood sample is drawn, you drink a solution containing 100 mg of glucose, following which blood is drawn every thirty minutes for two hours, and then every hour for four hours. This reveals how your body processes sugar. A level above 200 mg/dL may mean you have diabetes; if the level is the same on a second day, the diagnosis is confirmed.

A urine test can also be conducted to detect ketones (a by-product produced in diabetes, starvation, and dehydration). Ketones aren't used to diagnose diabetes, but the test can help guide insulin therapy.

Epilogue

Harry III was born on the eve of the new millennium, in the shadow of the once-fertile Ohio cornfields of his grandfather's farm. He is his father's son, with his grandfather's stoic soul. But Harry III's story has a different ending.

Abandoning the rich farm breakfasts of his forebears, Harry and his family eat many small meals featuring high-protein, low-fat foods. The fast-food chains that used to push animal fats to children are teaching Harry and his family how to eat right, and serve foods that not only taste great but also keep our blood thin. Fond of fish and accustomed to daily vitamins and exercise, at age twelve, Harry begins a monthly program of checking and documenting his physiologic functions using his home computer. He is thin and fit; his blood pressure is 90/60. Harry III feels the quickening of his pulse; he feels the exuberance of his own blood.

I am the aorta. The blood flows easily, like a gentle stream. I absorb the slow pulsations of the heart with ease. Life is peaceful, quiet. I am the aorta. And I have so much to live for . . .

By the year 2020, Harry III is a full-time computer programming student at the university. Isolated for hours on end in front of a flickering computer screen, Harry has abandoned his healthy lifestyle. His food cravings, even for the no-animal-fat Big Mac, have sent his weight soaring. His blood pressure has climbed to 110/90, a level once considered "normal" but, for Harry III, too high. At the same time, his doctor discovers that his blood is getting too thick and sticky.

I am the aorta. The blood flow is harder now. The insistent pulsating flow is stretching my overexpansion zone, just a little. The pressure increases. I must absorb the pressure . . . I keep stretching . . . and get a bit tougher.

Quickly observing his health problems, doctors implant a device in Harry's left shoulder to help him excrete excess blood fats into his urine for elimination. Another device is implanted in the artery of his wrist to monitor his blood pressure and heart contractility twenty-four hours a day. He begins donating a pint of blood each month, and taking 525 milligrams of aspirin daily which was tailored to his individualized care plan. The new treatments are successful. By age twenty-two, Harry is back to his normal weight. He starts on a new blood pressure medication that keeps his blood pressure no higher than 90/60 during *all* his daily activities.

In his early forties, Harry finishes his education and begins working in an auto levitation mobile manufacturing plant, in quality assurance. His stress levels are high: he has been married twice and has five children. He has hydrated himself with alcohol and cappuccino, and several new "street" drugs are causing an increase in his blood pressure and viscosity.

I am the aorta. My walls are thickening again. The stress is hurting me. Blood flow is pounding harder now. I can no longer stretch or bulge as easily with each beat.

Harry's monthly body tune-up shows that his cardiac injury index is increasing, so he begins taking medication to reduce his red blood cell age and decrease the stickiness of his blood. He starts donating blood again. A year later, his injury index has returned to normal.

I am the aorta. The blood is calm again, like the blood I knew when I was young. It's no longer sticky. It takes so little to move this fine and gentle blood, gliding smoothly around my branches. It doesn't stick or tear. I am becoming soft and supple once again. I welcome the incoming blood with my new elasticity. I am the aorta. I have so much to live for . . .

At age sixty, Harry is at his normal weight. He exercises regularly, keeps hydrated, eats many small meals, and has been cured of a bout with kidney cancer. The cancer was removed, and his kidney was replaced using an organ grown from his own kidney cells in a genetics lab. At seventy, Harry returns to school for a Ph.D. in mind therapy. He wants to make his mark on the world by exploring the last great unknown and trying to discover a cure for the soul. He sets out in search of it.

I am the aorta. And I have so much to live for . . .

The year is 2125, and at age 125, Harry enjoys playing a round of golf on the first golf course on the moon. It's getting crowded there, much like Earth. Harry moved here twenty years before to find some peace and quiet, but even now, life's becoming hectic.

I am Harry's arteries. No different from when I was twelve years old. I am soft and flexible; the blood moves gently by, with only slow pulsations of slippery, thin fluid gliding along my lining. I am happy. Life goes on with little effort.

Glossary

Aorta   The large artery that receives blood from the left ventricle of the heart and distributes it to the body.

Arrhythmia (Dysrhythmia)   An abnormal rhythm of the heart.

Artery   Any one of a series of vessels that carries blood from the heart to the various parts of the body.

Balloon angioplasty   A procedure in which a balloon is inserted into a narrowed area of a blood vessel. When the balloon is inflated, the narrowed area is stretched open and then the balloon is removed. Also called balloon dilation angioplasty.

Blood pressure   The force or pressure exerted by the heart in pumping blood; pressure of the blood in the arteries. It is maintained by the contraction of the left ventricle, the resistance of the arterioles and capillaries, the elasticity of the arterial walls, and the viscosity and volume of the blood.

Cardiac arrest   A condition in which the heart stops beating.

Cardiology   The study of the heart and its functions in health and disease.

Cardiovascular   Pertaining to the heart and blood vessels.

Catheterization   The process of examining the heart by inserting a thin tube (catheter) into a vein or artery and passing it into the heart. It's done to sample oxygen, measure pressure, and make x-ray movies.

Congestive heart failure   The inability of the heart to pump out all the blood that returns to it. This results in blood backing up in the veins that lead to the heart. Sometimes fluid builds up in various parts of the body.

Coronary arteries   Two arteries traveling from the aorta, arching down over the top of the heart, that provide blood to the heart muscle.

Diastolic blood pressure   The pressure inside the arteries when the heart muscle is relaxed.

Diuretic   A drug that increases the rate that urine forms, promoting the excretion of water and salts.

Dysrhythmia (Arrhythmia)   An abnormal rhythm of the heart.

Echocardiography   A diagnostic method in which pulses of sound are bounced off the surface of the heart and are plotted and recorded on electronic equipment.

Electrocardiogram (ECG or EKG)   A graphic record of electrical impulses produced by the heart.

Hypertension   The medical term for high blood pressure—a chronic increase in blood pressure above the normal range.

Pacemaker   An artificial pacemaker is an electrical device that controls the heart's beating and rhythm by emitting a series of electrical discharges.

Pulmonary artery   The large artery that receives blood from the right ventricle and takes it to the lungs.

Stent   A mechanical device placed in an artery to allow blood to flow through more easily. It acts to reduce the size of the plaque that is obstructing the artery.

Systolic blood pressure   The pressure inside the arteries when the heart contracts with each beat.

Ultrasound   High-frequency sound vibration that a human ear cannot hear, used in medical diagnosis. The ultrasound test includes both echocardiography to show a picture of the heart and a Doppler test that analyzes blood flow.

Valve   An opening, covered by membrane flaps, between two chambers of the heart or between a chamber of the heart and a blood vessel. When it's closed, no blood normally passes through.

Vascular   Pertaining to the blood vessels.

Vein   Any one of a series of vessels that carries blood from various parts of the body back to the heart.

Ventricle   One of the two lower chambers of the heart.

Viscosity   The thickness and resistance of a fluid.

Resources for More Information

Anxiety/Stress

American Institute of Stress
124 Park Ave.
New York, NY 10703
(914) 963-1200; (800) 24-RELAX

Anxiety Disorders Association of America
11900 Parklawn Dr., #100
Rockville, MD 20852
(301) 231-9350

International Stress Management Association
10455 Pomerado Rd.
San Diego, CA 92131
(619) 693-4698

Diabetes

American Diabetes Association
P.O. Box 25757
1660 Duke St.
Alexandria, VA 22314
(800) 342-2383

National Diabetes Information Clearinghouse
1 Information Way
Bethesda, MD 20892
(301) 654-3327

Diet

American Dietetic Association
216 W. Jackson Blvd.
Chicago, IL 60605
(312) 899-0040

Exercise

Aerobics and Fitness Association of America
15250 Ventura Blvd., Suite 200
Sherman Oaks, CA 91403
(800) 446-2322

American Council on Exercise
5820 Oberlin Dr., Suite 102
San Diego, CA 92121
(800) 825-3636
www.acefitness.org

President's Council on Physical Fitness and Sports
200 Independence Ave. SW
Hubert Humphrey Bldg., Room 738-H
Washington, DC 20201
(202) 690-9000

Heart Disease

American Heart Association
7320 Greenville Ave.
Dallas, TX 75231
(214) 373-6300
www.americanheart.org

American Medical Women's Association Education Project
   on Coronary Heart Disease in Women
801 N. Fairfax St., #400
Alexandria, VA 22314
(703) 838-0500

National Heart, Lung, and Blood Institute Information Center
P.O. Box 30105
Bethesda, MD 20824
(800) 575-WELL
www.nhlbi.nih.gov

Visco Technologies, Inc.
15 East Uwchlan Avenue
Suite 414
Exton, PA 19341
(800) 969-2585
www.viscotech.com

References

Chapter 1

Antonova, N., and Velcheva, I. "Hemorheological disturbances and characteristic parameters in patients with cerebrovascular disease." *Clinical Hemorheology and Microcirculation* 21, no. 3–4 (1999): 405–8.

Bonithon-Kopp, C., et al. "Longitudinal associations between plasma viscosity and cardiovascular risk factors in a middle-aged French population." *Atherosclerosis* 104, no. 1–2 (1993): 173–82.

Cho, Y. I., and K. R. Kensey. "Effects of the non-Newtonian viscosity of blood on flows in a diseased arterial vessel: Part I, Steady flows." *Biorheology* 28, no. 3–4 (1991): 241–62.

Chobanian, A. V. "The influence of hypertension and other hemodynamic factors in atherogenesis." *Progress in Cardiovascular Diseases* 26, no. 3 (1983): 177–96.

Gordon, T., and W. B. Kannel. "Predisposition to atherosclerosis in the head, heart, and legs. The Framingham Study." *Journal of the American Medical Association* 221, no. 7 (1972): 661–6.

Hopkins, P. N., and R. R. Williams. "A survey of 246 suggested coronary risk factors." *Atherosclerosis* 40 (1981): 1–52.

————. "Identification and relative weight of cardiovascular risk factors." *Cardiology Clinics* 4 (1986): 3–31.

Kensey, K. R., and Y. I. Cho. "A theory implicating protective adaptation to chronic mechanical injury as the etiology of arterial occlusive disease." *Journal of Invasive Cardiology* 6 (1994): 55–70.

Malek, A. M., S. L. Alper, and S. Izumo. "Hemodynamic shear stress and its role in atherosclerosis." *Journal of the American Medical Association* 282, no. 21 (1999): 2035–42.

Ross, R. "The pathogenesis of atherosclerosis—an update." *New England Journal of Medicine* 314, no. 8 (1986): 488–500.

Sloop, G. D. "A unifying theory of atherogenesis." *Medical Hypotheses* 47, no. 4 (1996): 321–5.

Wong, N., H. R. Black, and J. M. Gardin. *Preventive Cardiology.* New York: McGraw-Hill, 2000.

Yarnell, J. W. G., et al. "Lifestyle and hemostatic risk factors for ischemic heart disease: The Caerphilly Study." *Arteriosclerosis, Thrombosis, and Vascular Biology* 20, no. 1 (January 2000): 271–9.

Chapter 2

Cinar Y., et al. "Effect of hematocrit on blood pressure via hyperviscosity." *American Journal of Hypertension* 12, no. 7 (1999): 739–43.

Jiang, Y., K. Kohara, and K. Hiwada. "Low wall shear stress contributes to atherosclerosis of the carotid artery in hypertensive patients." *Hypertension Research* 22, no. 3 (1999): 203–7.

Joint National Committee on Prevention, Detection, Evaluation, and Treatment of High Blood Pressure. "The Sixth Report of the Joint National Committee on Prevention, Detection, Evaluation, and Treatment of High Blood Pressure." *Archives of Internal Medicine* 157, no. 21 (1997): 2413–46.

Khder, Y., et al. "Shear stress abnormalities contribute to endothelial dysfunction in hypertension but not in type II diabetes." *Journal of Hypertension* 16, no. 11 (1998): 1619–25.

MacMahon, S., et al. "Blood pressure, stroke, and coronary heart disease." *Lancet* 335, no. 8692 (1990): 765–74.

Poli, K. A., et al. "Association of blood pressure with fibrinolytic potential in the Framingham offspring population." *Circulation* 101, no. 3 (2000): 264–9.

Stamler, J., R. Stamler, and J. D. Neaton. "Blood pressure, systolic and diastolic, and cardiovascular risks. U.S. population data." *Archives of Internal Medicine* 153 (1993): 598–615.

Wong, N., H. R. Black, and J. M. Gardin. *Preventive Cardiology*. New York: McGraw-Hill, 2000.

Chapter 3

Carallo, C., et al. "Whole blood viscosity and haematocrit are associated with internal carotid atherosclerosis in men." *Coronary Artery Disease* 9, no. 2–3 (1998): 113–7.

Cicco, G., et al. "Hemorheology in complicated hypertension." *Clinical Hemorheology and Microcirculation* 21, no. 3–4 (1999): 315–9.

Cicco, G., and A. Pirrelli. "Red blood cell (RBC) deformability, RBC aggregability, and tissue oxygenation in hypertension." *Clinical Hemorheology and Microcirculation* 21, no. 3–4 (1999): 169–77.

Fowkes, F. G., et al. "Sex differences in susceptibility to etiologic factors for peripheral atherosclerosis; importance of plasma fibrinogen and blood viscosity." *Arteriosclerosis and Thrombosis* 14, no. 6 (June 1994): 862–8.

Fowkes, F. G., et al. "The relationship between blood viscosity and blood pressure in a random sample of the population aged 55 to 74 years." *European Heart Journal* 14, no. 5 (May 1993): 597–601.

Kensey, K. R., Y. I. Cho, and M. Chang. "Effects of whole blood viscosity on atherogenesis." *Journal of Invasive Cardiology* 9 (1997): 17–24.

Knight, P. K., S. P. Ray, and R. J. Rose. "Effects of phlebotomy and autologous blood transfusion on oxygen transport in the racehorse." *Equine Veterinary Journal Supplement* 30 (July 1999): 143–7.

Larsson, H., et al. "Studies on blood viscosity during the menstrual cycle and in the postmenopausal period in healthy women." *Acta Obstetricia et Gynecologica Scandinavica* 68 (1989): 483–6.

Lee, A. J., et al. "Blood viscosity and elevated carotid intima-media thickness in men and women: The Edinburgh Artery Study." *Circulation* 97, no. 15 (April 21, 1998): 1467–73.

Letcher, R. L., et al. "Direct relationship between blood pressure and blood viscosity in normal and hypertensive subjects; role of fibrinogen and concentration." *American Journal of Medicine* 70, no. 6 (June 1981): 1195–1202.

Lowe, G. D., et al. "Increased blood viscosity in young women using oral contraceptives." *American Journal of Obstetrics and Gynecology* 137, no. 7 (August 1, 1980): 840–2.

Lowe, G. D., et al. "Relation between extent of coronary artery disease and blood viscosity." *British Medical Journal* 280, no. 6215 (March 8, 1980): 673–4.

Ridker, P. M., et al. "C-reactive protein and other markers of inflammation in the prediction of cardiovascular disease in women." *New England Journal of Medicine* 342, no. 12 (March 23, 2000): 836–43.

Ridker, P. M., et al. "Prospective study of C-reactive protein and the risk of future cardiovascular events among apparently healthy women." *Circulation* 98, no. 8 (August 25, 1998): 731–3.

Rosenson, R. S., A. McCormick, and E. F. Uretz. "Distribution of blood viscosity values and biochemical correlates in healthy adults." *Clinical Chemistry* 42, no. 8 (August 1996): 1189–95.

Sandhagen, B. "Red cell fluidity in hypertension." *Clinical Hemorheology and Microcirculation* 21, no. 3–4 (1999): 179–81.

Chapter 4

Ajmani, R. S., and J. M. Rifkind. "Hemorheological changes during human aging." *Gerontology* 44, no. 2 (1998): 111–20.

de Simone, G., et al. "Relation of blood viscosity to demographic and physiologic variables and to cardiovascular risk factors in apparently normal adults." *Circulation* 81, no. 1 (1990): 107–17.

Ford, D. E., et al. "Depression is a risk factor for coronary artery disease in men: The Precursors Study." *Archives of Internal Medicine* 158, no. 13 (1998): 1422–6.

Gudmundsson, M., and A. Bjelle. "Plasma, serum and whole-blood viscosity variations with age, sex, and smoking habits." *Angiology* 44, (1993): 384–91.

Hamazaki, T., and H. Shishido. "Increase in blood viscosity due to alcohol drinking." *Thrombosis Research* 30, no. 6 (1983): 587–94.

Kiechl, S., et al. "Alcohol consumption and atherosclerosis: what is the relation? Prospective results from the Bruneck Study." *Stroke* 29, no. 5 (1998): 900–7.

McMillan, D. E. "Development of vascular complications in diabetes." *Vascular Medicine* 2, no. 2 (1997): 132–42.

Rampling, M. W. "Haemorheological disturbances in hypertension: The influence of diabetes and smoking." *Clinical Hemorheology and Microcirculation* 21, no. 3–4 (1999): 183–7.

Yarnell, J. W. G., et al. "Lifestyle and hemostatic risk factors for ischemic heart disease: The Caerphilly Study." *Ateriosclerosis, Thrombosis, and Vascular Biology* 20, no. 1 (January 2000): 271–9.

Chapter 5

Assmann, G., et al. "The emergence of triglycerides as a significant independent risk factor in coronary artery disease." *European Heart Journal* 19, Supplement M (1998): M8–14.

Crowley, J. P., et al. "Low density lipoprotein cholesterol and whole blood viscosity." *Annals of Clinical and Laboratory Science* 24 no. 6 (1994): 533–41.

Kummerow, F. A., et al. "The relationship of oxidized lipids to coronary artery stenosis." *Atherosclerosis*, 149, no. 1 (2000): 181–90.

Malinow, M. R., A. G. Bostom, and R. M. Krauss. "Homocyst(e)ine, diet, and cardiovascular diseases: A statement for healthcare professionals from the Nutrition Committee, American Heart Association." *Circulation* 99 (1999): 178–82.

Ridker, P. M., et al. "Homocysteine and risk of cardiovascular disease among postmenopausal women." *Journal of the American Medical Association* 281 (1999): 1817–21.

Rimm, E. B., et al. "Folate and vitamin B6 from diet and supplements in relation to risk of coronary heart disease among women." *Journal of the American Medical Association* 279 (1998): 359–64.

Sloop, G. D., and D. E. Mercante. "Opposite effects of low-density and high-density lipoprotein on blood viscosity in fasting subjects." *Clinical Hemorheology and Microcirculation* 19, no. 3 (1998): 197–203.

Verhoef, P., et al. "Plasma total homocysteine, B vitamins, and risk of coronary atherosclerosis." *Arteriosclerosis, Thrombosis, and Vascular Biology* 17 (1997): 989–95.

Chapter 6

Clivillé, X., et al. "Hemorheological, coagulative and fibrinolytic changes during autologous blood donation." *Clinical Hemorheology and Microcirculation* 18, no. 4 (1998): 265–72.

Kameneva, M. V., et al. "Red blood cell aging and risk of cardiovascular diseases." *Clinical Hemorheology and Microcirculation* 18 (1998): 67–74.

Kameneva, M. V., M. J. Watach, and H. S. Borovetz. "Gender difference in rheologic properties of blood and risk of cardiovascular diseases." *Clinical Hemorheology and Microcirculation* 21, no. 3–4 (1999): 357–63.

Meyers, D. G., et al. "Possible association of a reduction in cardiovascular events with blood donation." *Heart* 78, no. 2 (1997): 188–93.

Samsioe, G. "Cardiovascular disease in postmenopausal women." *Maturitas* 30, no. 1 (September 20, 1998): 11–8.

Tremollieres, F. A., et al. "Coronary heart disease risk factors and menopause: A study in 1,684 French women." *Atherosclerosis* 142, no. 2 (February 1999): 415–23.

Tuomainen, T. P., et al. "Cohort study of relation between donating blood and risk of myocardial infarction in 2682 men in eastern Finland." *British Medical Journal* 314, no. 7083 (1997): 793–4.

Chapter 7

Husain, S., et al. "Aspirin improves endothelial dysfunction in atherosclerosis." *Circulation* 97, no. 8 (1998): 716–20.

Ikonomidis, I., et al. "Increased proinflammatory cytokines in patients with chronic stable angina and their reduction by aspirin." *Circulation* 100, no. 8 (1999): 793–8.

Kodama, M., et al. "Antiplatelet drugs attenuate progression of carotid intima-media thickness in subjects with type 2 diabetes." *Thrombosis Research* 97, no. 4 (2000): 239–45.

Pernerstorfer, T., et al. "Low-dose aspirin does not lower in vivo platelet activation in healthy smokers." *British Journal of Haematology* 102, no. 5 (1998): 1229–31.

Ross, R. "Atherosclerosis—an inflammatory disease." *New England Journal of Medicine* 340, no. 2 (1999): 115–26.

Sloop, G. D. "Decreased prevalence of symptomatic atherosclerosis in arthritis patients on long-term aspirin therapy." *Angiology* 49, no. 10 (1998): 827–32.

Chapter 8

Blann, A., A. Bignell, and C. McCollum. "Von Willebrand factor, fibrinogen, and other plasma proteins as determinants of plasma viscosity." *Atherosclerosis* 139, no. 2 (1998): 317–22.

Fiscella, K., and P. Franks. "Cost-effectiveness of the transdermal nicotine patch as an adjunct to physicians' smoking cessation counseling." *Journal of the American Medical Association* 275, no. 16 (1996): 1247–51.

Gudmundsson, M., and A. Bjelle. "Plasma, serum, and whole-blood viscosity variations with age, sex, and smoking habits." *Angiology* 44 (1993): 384–91.

Lowe, G. D. "Etiopathogenesis of cardiovascular disease: Hemostasis, thrombosis, and vascular medicine." *Annals of Periodontology* 3, no. 1 (1998): 121–6.

Lowe, G. D., et al. "The effects of age and cigarette-smoking on blood and plasma viscosity in men." *Scottish Medical Journal* 25, no. 1 (January 1980): 13–7.

Masson, C. L., and D. G. Gilbert. "Cardiovascular and mood responses to quantified doses of cigarette smoke in oral contraceptive users and nonusers." *Journal of Behavioral Medicine* 22, no. 6 (December 1999): 589–604.

McCarty, M. F. "Interleukin-6 as a central mediator of cardiovascular risk associated with chronic inflammation, smoking, diabetes, and visceral obesity: Down-regulation with essential fatty acids, ethanol, and pentoxifylline." *Medical Hypotheses* 52, no. 5 (1999): 465–77.

Price, J. F., et al. "Relationship between smoking and cardiovascular risk factors in the development of peripheral arterial disease and coronary artery disease: Edinburgh Artery Study." *European Heart Journal* 20, no. 5 (March 1999): 344–53.

Rothwell, M., et al. "Haemorheological changes in the very short term after abstention from tobacco by cigarette smokers." *British Journal of Haematology* 79, no. 3 (1991): 500–3.

Smith, F. B., et al. "Smoking, hemorheologic factors, and progression of peripheral arterial disease in patients with claudication." *Journal of Vascular Surgery* 28, no. 1 (July 1998): 129–35.

Yarnell, J. W. G., et al. "Lifestyle and hemostatic risk factors for ischemic heart disease: The Caerphilly Study." *Arteriosclerosis, Thrombosis, and Vascular Biology* 20, no. 1 (January 2000): 271–9.

Chapter 9

Baraona, E., and C. S. Lieber. "Alcohol and lipids." *Recent Developments in Alcoholism* 14 (1998): 97–134.

Cinar, Y., et al. "Effect of hematocrit on blood pressure via hyperviscosity." *American Journal of Hypertension* 12, no. 7 (1999): 739–43.

Galea, G., and R. J. Davidson. "Some haemorheological and haematological effects of alcohol." *Scandinavian Journal of Haematology* 30, no. 4 (1983): 308–10.

Hamazaki, T., and H. Shishido. "Increase in blood viscosity due to alcohol drinking." *Thrombosis Research* 30, no. 6 (1983): 587–94.

Hillbom, M. E., et al. "Effect of ethanol on blood viscosity and erythrocyte flexibility in healthy men." *European Journal of Clinical Investigation* 13, no. 1 (1983): 45–8.

Kiechl, S., et al. "Alcohol consumption and atherosclerosis: What is the relation? Prospective results from the Bruneck Study." *Stroke* 29, no. 5 (1998): 900–7.

Oonishi, T., and K. Sakashita. "Ethanol improves decreased filterability of human red blood cells through modulation of intracellular signaling pathways." *Alcoholism, Clinical and Experimental Research* 24, no. 3 (2000): 352–6.

Puddey, I. B., et al. "Alcohol, free radicals, and antioxidants." *Novartis Foundation Symposium* 216 (1998): 51–62.

van de Weil, A. "Alcohol and insulin sensitivity." *Netherlands Journal of Medicine* 52, no. 3 (1998): 91–4.

van Tol, A., et al. "Changes in postprandial lipoproteins of low and high density caused by moderate alcohol consumption with dinner." *Atherosclerosis* 141, Supplement 1 (1998): S101–3.

Chapter 10

Albert, C. M., et al. "Fish consumption and risk of sudden cardiac death." *Journal of the American Medical Association* 279 (1998): 23–8.

Anthony, M. S., T. B. Clarkson, and J. K. Williams. "Effects of soy isoflavones on atherosclerosis: potential mechanisms." *American Journal of Clinical Nutrition* 68, Supplement 6 (1998): 1390–3S.

Armellini, F., et al. "Body fat distribution and whole blood viscosity in a sample of Italian men and women." *American Journal of Cardiology* 74 (1994): 200–2.

Israel, D. H., and R. Gorlin. "Fish oils in the prevention of atherosclerosis." *Journal of the American College of Cardiology* 19 (1992): 174–85.

Kinsella, J. E. "Effects of polyunsaturated fatty acids on factors related to cardiovascular disease." *American Journal of Cardiology* 60, no. 12 (1987): 23–32G.

Malinow, M. R., A. G. Bostom, and R. M. Krauss. "Homocyst(e)ine, diet, and cardiovascular diseases: A statement for healthcare professionals from the Nutrition Committee, American Heart Association." *Circulation* 99 (1999): 178–82.

McCarty, M. F. "Interleukin-6 as a central mediator of cardiovascular risk associated with chronic inflammation, smoking, diabetes, and visceral obesity: Down-regulation with essential fatty acids, ethanol, and pentoxifylline." *Medical Hypotheses* 52, no. 5 (1999): 465–77.

Messina, M. "Modern applications for an ancient bean: soybeans and the prevention and treatment of chronic disease." *Journal of Nutrition* 125, Supplement 3 (1995): 567–9S.

Ridker, P. M. et al. "Homocysteine and risk of cardiovascular disease among postmenopausal women." *Journal of the American Medical Association* (281): 1999, 1817–21.

Rimm, E. B., et al. "Folate and vitamin B6 from diet and supplements in relation to risk of coronary heart disease among women." *Journal of the American Medical Association* 279 (1998): 359–64.

Serrano Rios, M. "Relationship between obesity and the increased risk of major complications in non-insulin-dependent diabetes mellitus." *European Journal of Clinical Investigation* 28, Supplement 2 (1998): 14–17.

Solerte, S. B., et al. "Hyperviscosity and microproteinuria in central obesity: Relevance to cardiovascular risk." *International Journal of Obesity and Related Metabolic Disorders* 21, no. 6 (1997): 417–23.

United States Department of Agriculture and United States Department of Health and Human Services. "Nutrition and your health: Dietary guidelines for Americans." *Home and Garden Bulletin* no. 232. Fifth edition (2000).

Verhoef, P., et al. "Plasma total homocysteine, B vitamins, and risk of coronary atherosclerosis." *Arteriosclerosis, Thrombosis, and Vascular Biology* 17 (1997): 989–95.

Wilcox, J. N., and B. F. Blumenthal. "Thrombotic mechanisms in atherosclerosis: Potential impact of soy proteins." *Journal of Nutrition* 125, Supplement 3 (1995): 631–8S.

Yarnell, J. W. G., et al. "Lifestyle and hemostatic risk factors for ischemic heart disease: The Caerphilly Study." *Arteriosclerosis, Thrombosis, and Vascular Biology* 20, no. 1 (January 2000): 271–9.

Chapter 11

Benhaddad, A., et al. "Early hemorheologic aspects of overtraining in elite athletes." *Clinical Hemorheology and Microcirculation* 20, no. 2 (1999): 117–25.

Borst, M. M., et al. "Repetitive hemodilution in chronic obstructive pulmonary disease and pulmonary hypertension: Effects on pulmonary hemodynamics, gas exchange, and exercise capacity." *Respiration* 66, no. 3 (1999): 225–32.

Bouix, D., et al. "Fibrinogen is negatively correlated with aerobic working capacity in football players." *Clinical Hemorheology and Microcirculation* 19, no. 3 (1998): 219–27.

Bouix, D., et al. "Relationships among body composition, hemorheology, and exercise performance in rugbymen." *Clinical Hemorheology and Microcirculation* 19, no. 3 (1998): 245–54.

Brun, J. F., et al. "The triphasic effects of exercise on blood rheology: Which relevance to physiology and pathophysiology?" *Clinical Hemorheology and Microcirculation* 19, no. 2 (1998): 89–104.

Carroll, S., C. B. Cooke, and R. J. Butterly. "Physical activity, cardiorespiratory fitness, and the primary components of blood viscosity." *Medicine and Science in Sports and Exercise* 32, no. 2 (2000): 353–8.

El-Sayed, M. S. "Effects of exercise and training on blood rheology." *Sports Medicine* 26, no. 5 (1998): 281–92.

Galletta, F., et al. "Atherosclerosis vascular damage in elderly athletes and sedentary people." *Angiology* 48, no. 7 (1997): 623–8.

Khaled, S., et al. "Increased blood viscosity in iron-depleted elite athletes." *Clinical Hemorheology and Microcirculation* 18, no. 4 (1998): 309–18.

Reinhart, W. H., et al. "Influence of exercise training on blood viscosity in patients with coronary artery disease and impaired left ventricular function." *American Heart Journal* 135, no. 3 (1998): 379–82.

Wood, S. C., M. P. Doyle, and O. Appenzeller. "Effects of endurance training and long distance running on blood viscosity." *Medicine and Science in Sports and Exercise* 23 (1991): 1265–9.

Chapter 12

Broadwell, S. D., and K. C. Light. "Family support and cardiovascular responses in married couples during conflict and other interactions." *International Journal of Behavioral Medicine* 6, no. 1 (1999): 40–63.

Ford, D. E., et al. "Depression is a risk factor for coronary artery disease in men: The Precursors Study." *Archives of Internal Medicine* 158, no. 13 (July 13, 1998): 1422–26.

Frasure-Smith N., F. Lesperance, and M. Talajic. "Depression following myocardial infarction: Impact on six-month survival." *Journal of the American Medical Association* 270, no. 15 (1993): 1819–25.

Friedman, M., et al. "Effect of type A behavioral counseling on frequency of episodes of silent myocardial ischemia in coronary patients." *American Heart Journal* 132, no. 5 (November 1996): 933–7.

Kamarck, T. W. et al. "Exaggerated blood pressure responses during mental stress are associated with enhanced carotid atherosclerosis in middle-aged Finnish men: Findings from the Kuopio Ischemic Heart Disease Study." *Circulation* 96, no. 11 (December 2, 1997): 3843–8.

Kawachi, I., et al. "Prospective study of a self-report type A scale and risk of coronary heart disease: Test of the MMPI-2 type A scale." *Circulation* 98, no. 5 (August 4, 1998): 405–12.

Penninx, B. W., et al. "Cardiovascular events and mortality in newly and chronically depressed persons >70 years of age." *American Journal of Cardiology* 81, no. 8 (April 15, 1998): 988–94.

Rozanski, A., J. A. Blumenthal, and J. Kaplan. "Impact of psychological factors on the pathogenesis of cardiovascular disease and implications for therapy." *Circulation* 99, no. 16 (April 27, 1999): 2192–217.

Yudkin, J. S., et al. "Inflammation, obesity, stress, and coronary heart disease: Is interleukin-6 the link?" *Atherosclerosis* 148, no. 2 (2000): 209–14.

Chapter 13

Bass, J. A., T. Moore, and K. J. Stewart. "Coronary heart disease risk factors in children and adolescents." *Preventive Cardiology* 19 (1999): 112–7.

Berenson, G. S., et al. "Association between multiple cardiovascular risk factors and atherosclerosis in children and young adults: The Bogalusa Heart Study." *New England Journal of Medicine* 338 (1998): 1650–6.

Elkasabany, A. M., et al. "Prediction of adult hypertension by K4 and K5 diastolic blood pressure in children: The Bogalusa Heart Study." *Journal of Pediatrics* 132 (1998): 687–92.

Fox, B., et al. "Distribution of fatty and fibrous plaques in young human carotid arteries." *Atherosclerosis* 41 (1982): 337–47.

Hohn, A. R., K. M. Dwyer, and J. H. Dwyer. "Blood pressure in youth from four ethnic groups: The Pasadena Prevention Project." *Journal of Pediatrics* 125 (1994): 368–73.

Lauer, R. M., and W. R. Clarke. "Use of cholesterol measurements in childhood for the prediction of adult hypercholesterolemia." *Journal of the American Medical Association* 264 (1990): 3034–8.

Liu, K., et al. "Blood pressure in young blacks and whites; relevance of obesity and lifestyle factors in determining differences: The CARDIA Study." *Circulation* 93 (1996): 60–6.

Masson, C. L., and D. G. Gilbert. "Cardiovascular and mood responses to quantified doses of cigarette smoke in oral contraceptive users and nonusers." *Journal of Behavioral Medicine* 22, no. 6 (December 1999): 589–604.

National High Blood Pressure Education Program Working Group on Hypertension Control in Children and Adolescents. "Update on the 1987 Task Force Report on high blood pressure in children and adolescents: A working group report from the National High Blood Pressure Education Program." *Pediatrics* 98 (1996): 649–58.

Newman, W. P., W. Wattigney, and G. S. Berenson. "Autopsy studies in United States children and adolescents: Relationship of risk factors to atherosclerotic lesions." *Annals of the New York Academy of Science* 623 (1991): 16–25.

Stewart, K. J., et al. "Physical fitness, physical activity, and fatness in relation to blood pressure and lipids in preadolescent children: Results from the FRESH Study." *Journal of Cardiopulmonary Rehabilitation* 15 (1995): 122–9.

Stewart, K. J., and A. P. Goldberg. "Exercise, lipids, and obesity in adolescents with parental history of coronary disease." *American Journal of Health Promotion* 6, no. 6 (1992): 430–6.

Stewart, K. J., et al. "Dietary fat and cholesterol intake in young children compared with recommended levels." *Journal of Cardiopulmonary Rehabilitation* 19, no. 2 (1999): 112–7.

Strong, J. P., et al. "Prevalence and extent of atherosclerosis in adolescents and young adults: Implications for prevention from the Pathobiological Determinants of Atherosclerosis in Youth Study." *Journal of the American Medical Association* 281 (1999): 727–35.

Van Horn, L., and P. Greenland. "Prevention of coronary artery disease is a pediatric problem." *Journal of the American Medical Association* 278 (1997): 1779–80.

Wattigney, W. A., et al. "The emergence of clinically abnormal levels of cardiovascular disease risk factor variables among young adults: The Bogalusa Heart Study." *Preventive Medicine* 24 (1995): 617–26.

Webber, L. S., et al. "Cardiovascular risk factors among third grade children in four regions of the United States: The CATCH Study." *American Journal of Epidemiology* 141 (1995): 428–39.

Chapter 14

Ajmani, R. S., and J. M. Rifkind. "Hemorheological changes during human aging." *Gerontology* 44, no. 2 (1998): 111–20.

Ali, S. S., and J. R. Sowers. "Update on the management of hypertension; treatment of the elderly and diabetic hypertensives: Is the approach to management really different?" *Cardiovascular Reviews and Report* 6 (1998): 44–46, 51–54.

American Diabetes Association. "Aspirin therapy in diabetes." *Diabetes Care* 20, no. 11 (1997): 1772–3.

Clarkson, P., et al. "Impaired vascular reactivity in insulin-dependent diabetes mellitus is related to disease duration and low-density lipoprotein cholesterol levels." *Journal of the American College of Cardiology* 28 (1996): 573–9.

Fujisawa, T., et al. "Association of plasma fibrinogen level and blood pressure with diabetic retinopathy, and renal complications associated with proliferative diabetic retinopathy, in Type 2 diabetes mellitus." *Diabetic Medicine* 16, no. 6 (1999): 522–6.

Kannel, W. B., and D. L. McGee. "Diabetes and cardiovascular disease: The Framingham Study." *Journal of the American Medical Association* 241 (1979): 2035–8.

Komatsu, R., N. Tsushima, and T. Matsuyama. "Effects of glucagon administration on microcirculation and blood rheology." *Clinical Hemorheology and Microcirculation* 17, no. 4 (1997): 271–7.

Manson, J. E., et al. "A prospective study of maturity-onset diabetes mellitus and risk of coronary heart disease and stroke in women." *Archives of Internal Medicine* 151 (1991): 1141–7.

McCarty, M. F. "Interleukin-6 as a central mediator of cardiovascular risk associated with chronic inflammation, smoking, diabetes, and visceral obesity: Down-regulation with essential fatty acids, ethanol, and pentoxifylline." *Medical Hypotheses* 52, no. 5 (1999): 465–77.

McMillan, D. E. "Development of vascular complications in diabetes." *Vascular Medicine* 2, no. 2 (1997): 132–42.

Mellinghoff, A. C., et al. "Influence of glycemic control on viscosity and density of plasma and whole blood in Type I diabetic patients." *Diabetes Research and Clinical Practice* 33, no. 2 (1996): 75–82.

Persson, S. U., H. Larsson, and H. Odeberg. "Reduced number of circulating monocytes after institution of insulin therapy: Relevance for development of atherosclerosis in diabetics?" *Angiology* 49, no. 6 (1998): 423–33.

Ruige, J. B., et al. "Insulin and risk of cardiovascular disease: A meta-analysis." *Circulation* 97, no. 10 (1998): 996–1001.

Sagel, J., et al. "Increased platelet aggregation in early diabetes mellitus." *Annals of Internal Medicine* 82, no. 6 (1975): 733–8.

Schaefer, E. J., et al. "Lipoprotein (a) levels and risk of coronary heart disease in men." *Journal of the American Medical Association* 271, no. 13 (1994): 999–1003.

Serrano Rios, M. "Relationship between obesity and the increased risk of major complications in non-insulin-dependent diabetes mellitus." *European Journal of Clinical Investigation* 28, Supplement 2 (1998): 14–7.

Solerte, S. B., and M. Fioravanti. "Hemodynamic alterations in long-term insulin-dependent diabetic patients with overt hephropathy: Role of blood hyperviscosity and plasma protein changes." *Clinical Nephrology* 28, no. 3 (1987): 138–43.

Sowers, J. R. "Diabetes mellitus and cardiovascular disease in women." *Archives of Internal Medicine* 158, no. 6 (1998): 617–21.

Sowers, J. R., and M. A. Lester. "Diabetes and cardiovascular disease." *Diabetes Care*, Supplement 3 (1999): C14–20.

Wingard, D. L., and E. Barrett-Connor. "Heart disease and diabetes." In *Diabetes in America*. 2nd ed. Bethesda, Md.: National Institutes of Health (Pub. #95-1468), 1995.

Wingard, D. L., E. L. Barrett-Connor, and A. Ferrara. "Is insulin really a heart disease risk factor?" *Diabetes Care* 18, no. 9 (1995): 1299–304.

Index